Depression Since Prozac
Finding the True Self

for O.J. and Kathleen

Depression Since Prozac
Finding the True Self

Russell Helms

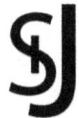

copyright © 2025, Russell Helms

sij books
PO BOX 4945
Chattanooga, TN 37405

sijbooks.com

Please inquire for rights to duplicate material in this book.

Printed in the Unites States of America

First edition

ISBN: 978-1-943661-45-9

Cover photo by Yoal Desurmont

Contents

Prozac: An Argument for Authenticity	1
Suicide	2
Getting Diagnosed	4
Prozac to the Rescue	4
The Rudiments of Depression	6
Prozac Nation	7
Prozac Diary	10
Artificial Happiness	11
Better than Well	14
The True Self	20
What is Depression?	27
The Severity and Spread of Depression	38
The Cost of Depression	41
Are We Happy Yet?	45
The *World Happiness Report*	49
A Short History of Depression	52
Asylums and Enlightenment	53
The Twentieth Century	59
The First Antidepressants	64
Antipsychiatry	65
The Revival of Biological Psychiatry	67
Sweet Serotonin	71
Side Effects of Increasing Serotonin	76
Sexual Dysfunction	77
The Rise of Prozac	79
The Cost of Prozac	87
The Diagnostic and Statistical Manual of Mental Disorders	89

Prozac Today	94
Prozac Under Fire	97
The Placebo Effect	97
Antidepressants and Children and Teenagers	101
Prozac and Violence	105
Marketing Antidepressants	109
Prozac and Creativity	120
Suicide	134
Therapy versus Antidepressants	146
Cognitive Behavioral Therapy	147
Psychoanalysis	151
Depression Since Prozac—Final Words	155
References	162

Prozac: An Argument for Authenticity

Does taking Prozac winnow away that sadness that is so dear to life, so essential, some say, rendering one inauthentic? Are we to maintain the true self at all costs, foregoing treatment in an effort to avoid falsity? Could the medicated self actually be the true self? Ultimately, depression is nasty. Depression kills, and any assuaging of its despair is not to be taken lightly, regardless of worries over authenticity.

Depression, whether mild, moderate, or severe, is a crippling disorder. According to the World Health Organization (WHO), more than 300 million people worldwide suffer from depression, and depression is the leading global cause of disability [1]. Generally, more women than men are affected, whites have higher rates of depression than blacks and Hispanics, and the poor are more depressed than the rich [2]. According to the Centers for Disease Control and Prevention (CDC), depression is associated with an increased risk of suicide, lower workplace productivity, other mental disorders such as anxiety, and even smoking [3].

The problem of depression is widespread. In 2015, an estimated 16.1 million United States adults 18 and older experienced at least one major depressive episode in the past year, representing 6.7 percent of all adults [4]. Looking at this in terms of happiness, according to the Pew Research Center, a third of adults in the United States say they're "very happy," another half say they are "pretty happy," and the rest consider themselves "not too happy" [2]. For casual purposes, we can identify unhappiness as a condition of life and depression as an illness, although the two bleed into one another.

Happiness on a global scale has been measured by Helliwell et al. using the World Happiness Report [5]. The United States ranks number thirteen, with Norway ranking highest in happiness, although the difference between the two is not statistically significant. It is interesting to note that eight of the bottom ten countries, the unhappiest of all, are in Africa. Faced with civil wars, famine, drought, pestilence, and disease, it is not hard to imagine being unhappy under such circumstances. It is estimated that 500,000 to 1 million people died in the Ethiopian famine of 1983 to 1986. In 1988, researchers in Ethiopia found that women in Addis Ababa, 94 out of a sample of 113, were suffering from what the women described as "oppression of the soul," something equivalent to chronic depression [6].

In terms of cost in the United States, the burden of depression, including workplace costs, direct costs, and suicide-related costs, was estimated to be $210.5 billion in 2010 [3]. Medications like Prozac are, of course, a substantial portion of this disease cost. According to Nassir Ghaemi, psychiatric medicine costs are only bested by cardiology drugs, which are used to treat the number one cause of mortality, heart disease [7].

Suicide

A touchstone of depression is suicide, the tragic consequence of a treatable disease's ultimate finality. Heart disease and cancer consistently rank as the number one and number two contributors to mortality. And also consistently, suicide comes in tenth place, which is hard to fathom. Even more alarming, suicide is the second leading cause of death among those aged 15–24 years, the second among persons aged 25-34 years, and the fourth among persons aged 35–54 [8]. In 2016, the CDC reported that more than 40,000 people died by suicide, more than 1 million people reported making a suicide attempt in the past year, and more than 2 million adults reported thinking about suicide in the past year [9]. Worldwide, it is estimated that 800,000 people per year take their lives [10]. To illuminate that statistic, worldwide every 40 seconds someone commits suicide, and many more attempt suicide [10].

And, suicide rates have continued to climb. According to the WHO, suicide deaths increased from 11.5 per 100,000 people in 1970 to 11.8 per 100,000 in 1980. By 1990, four years after the introduction of Prozac, the U.S. suicide death rate actually increased [11]. The CDC reports that from 1999 through 2014, the suicide rate in the United States increased 24 percent [12]. For the latest year available, 2015, 44,000 people in the United States died from suicide, which does not include accidental deaths that may have been masked suicides [13].

It is commonly thought that suicidal thoughts should improve as the depression improves, but there have been claims that medications such as Prozac actually increase suicidal thoughts [14]. One explanation is that the seriously depressed are too weak to carry out a plan of suicide and, once under treatment, but not fully controlled, the energy to carry out a suicide emerges. It is thus essential for depressed patients undergoing new treatment to be closely monitored and made aware of such a possibility. A "black box warning" issued in 2004 by the Food and Drug Administration disclosed the possibility of suicidal ideation. The warning stated that there was an increased risk of suicide in children and adolescents treated with medications like Prozac. In 2006, the warning was extended to young adults [15]. As a result, as reported by NBC News, many of those taking Prozac and similar antidepressants, including children with worried parents, quit the medications, leaving them untreated and vulnerable, possibly leading to the increase in suicides [16].

Getting Diagnosed

To be properly diagnosed with depression, or major depressive disorder, according to the American Psychiatric Association (APA), a person must experience five or more symptoms from the list below for a continuous period of at least two weeks:

- Feelings of sadness, hopelessness, depressed mood
- Loss of interest or pleasure in activities that used to be enjoyable
- Change in weight or appetite (either increase or decrease)
- Change in activity: psychomotor agitation (being more active
- than usual) or psychomotor retardation (being less active than usual)
- Insomnia (difficulty sleeping) or sleeping too much
- Feeling tired or not having any energy
- Feelings of guilt or worthlessness
- Difficulties concentrating and paying attention
- Thoughts of death or suicide

The CDC notes that symptoms should be present every day or nearly every day and should lead to significant distress [3]. In the twentieth century, diagnosing depression moved from a pseudo-science based on psychoanalysis to this research-based list of criteria now contained in the *Diagnostic and Statistical Manual of Mental Illness,* which is now in its fifth edition.

Prozac to the Rescue

Released in December 1987 was Eli Lilly's Prozac, a drug designed to increase the amount of serotonin in the brain. An SSRI, or selective serotonin reuptake inhibitor, Prozac blocks the reabsorption of serotonin within brain synapses once it has been released as a signaling agent. Interbrand, a leading global branding company, created the name Prozac. The name has been key in its success, indicating qualities of "positive, professional, quick, proey, zaccy" [17]. After testing Prozac with a variety of disorders, it was found to work with mild depression and was soon giving Eli Lilly, Prozac's maker, more than 25 percent of its $10 billion annual revenue [17].

Prozac and medications like it soared. By 1990, psychiatric patients receiving prescriptions increased from 25 percent of all office visits in 1975 to 50 percent by 1990 [18]. Also, depression as a diagnosis more than doubled between 1991 and 2001 [17]. This could very well be the case of a drug seeking its diagnosis, and certainly plays to the media attention given to depression since the release of Prozac. However, and unfortunately, we must remember that one in five Americans has a mental health condition, but only half receive mental health services [19].

According to the CDC, the percentage of the population prescribed Prozac and other antidepressants rose three-hundred-fold from 1988 to 2012 [20]. Although physicians were looking harder for depression, a new openness to depression, as evidenced by the rise in popular literature associated with Prozac, made people feel more comfortable admitting that they were depressed and were thus more willing to seek treatment and take medication.

Prozac was the first drug of its kind to gain a popular following, but there have been other medications that have created an allegiance. Chloral hydrate first appeared in Germany in 1832 and was widely popular as a hypnotic. Chloral hydrate foreshadowed the Prozac scenario, acquiring a great public following for relief from a mental illness [18]. Later, similar blockbuster scenarios occurred with the tranquilizer Miltown in 1955 and its successor Valium in the 1960s, 70s, and 80s.

In conjunction with the newness of depression as a more or less common disorder was a new phenomenon, depression emerging within popular literature, most notably Elizabeth

Wurtzel's *Prozac Nation*, which set off two decades of popular texts aimed at supporting and vilifying the enhancement qualities of SSRIs such as Prozac and bemoaning the loss of one's identity.

This deluge of media discussing Prozac and medications like it was unprecedented and a testament to the wonder and controversy surrounding Prozac.

The Rudiments of Depression

So, what is depression more fully, beyond the clinical view espoused by the APA? The writer William Styron describes depression from his gut using concrete language. Perhaps it was his memoir published in 1990 that really got the depression train moving. Styron notes "...the ferocious inwardness of the pain..." [21]. He also notes that the "...failure of alleviation is one of the most distressing factors of the disorder..." [21], which is very true in the absence of effective treatment with medications such as Prozac or through psychological intervention or both. Even staunch anti-Prozac writer Charles Barber says this: "Truly depressed people shake physically, are unable to get out of bed, and exude a profound heaviness or lifelessness, exhibiting a sort of death in life" [22]. Psychiatrist David Kramer, perhaps the lion of Prozac use, says that depression is "a progressive, probably lifelong disorder" [23]. Kramer even advocates that once treated for depression, the treatment should be lifelong as well. From Goethe's *The Sorrows of Young Werther*, we have this prescient text: "The leaven which animated my existence is gone: the charm which cheered me in the gloom of night, and aroused me from my morning slumbers, is forever fled" [24]. Was it better for Young Werther to suffer than to be helped?

Many answer that it is necessary to distinguish sadness from depression, thinking that sadness is a noble human characteristic that is dangerous to take away. According to Joseph Glenmullen,

"Genuine sadness is quite different from depression. Sadness is a clarifying, relieving emotion that helps one move on after losses" [25]. Eric Wilson thinks of sadness and depression as a continuum: "Of course, there is a fine line between what I'm calling melancholia and what society calls depression. In my mind, what separates the two is degree of activity" [26].

Depression is serious. Think about suicide, perhaps sadness gone askew. So, does sadness alone induce suicidal ideation? Perhaps not, but if the sadness has bled into the realm of extreme sadness, then we can label that as depression, which is deserving of treatment. However, sadness should be viewed as a symptom of depression, versus being within its own sterile category. When Wurtzel says, "So as far as I'm concerned, the last shower I took is the last shower I will ever take" [27], then we all need to be worried. Sylvia Plath said a similar thing about washing her hair, the futility. She would only have to repeat the motion, and what is the good of that, a despair of life in total.

Why do some people get depressed while others do not? Barber's answer is that "Psychiatric disorders are almost certainly the dialectical product of an infinitely complex dialogue between genes and the environment" [22]. Norden expounds on the environment, finding fault with the stress of modern society: "These cumulative stresses of modern life have set off an avalanche of depression, anxiety, and insomnia" [28]. Considering life's rough patches, Kramer adds that "People don't have to be made vulnerable by trauma: they can be born vulnerable" [23]. And ultimately, the crux of an argument for antidepressants is that depression "ruins...lives" [27].

Prozac Nation

We now turn to that famous book, adapted into an equally infamous movie, *Prozac Nation,* by Elizabeth Wurtzel, which says that "the deeply depressed are just the walking, waking dead" [27]. She gives us vivid accounts of what it is like to be seriously depressed. For example, "I walked away from Ruby, lost in vertigo. The Yard seemed like a phantom. I moved through it in the plastic bubble that separated my fogworld from everything around me" [27]. She gives us the effect of depression on setting, giving dead life to inanimate objects with flair.

In addition to the lifelessness of person and place, Wurtzel recounts what is most oppressive about depression, the debilitation of the routine. She says, "While I was still in my old room at home, I discovered that the hardest part of each day, as is the case with most depressives, was simply getting out of bed in the morning. If I could do that much, I had a fighting chance" [27]. Who wouldn't want to take a magic pill to try and soften the edges of such a burdened reality?

Once prescribed Prozac, Wurtzel finds that she has found her legs, has discovered her lot in life, as if her disease were some great egg that needed cracking. "Enter Prozac, and suddenly I have a diagnosis" [27]. And this is where the suffering can come to not an end, but at least to some resolution. Spending one's day like the "walking wounded" and "constantly embroiled in thoughts of suicide" is a quick way to spoil the human experience [27]. Interestingly, Wurtzel embraces her diagnosis, coming to know her depression more intimately as if it were an old friend who needed a push and a hug. "I had fallen in love with my depression...I loved it because I thought it was all I had" [27].

So, what happened to Wurtzel once she began her regimen of Prozac? A small miracle. She says, "And then something just kind of changed in me. Over the next few days, I became all right, safe in my own skin. It happened just like that" [27]. The miracle cure, a waning of the dead thoughts, a realization that one's love affair with depression was actually a dance with death. Once released from the claws of depression, we gain insight. Are we afraid of such a transformation? But Wurtzel is pragmatic, acknowledging that Prozac is "about the mainstreaming of mental illness in general and depression in particular" [27]. Prozac had made it possible to not only talk about depression but to embrace it.

So, what does Wurtzel think about the idea that the brain's unsalted soup is perhaps the real culprit, that boosting one's serotonin levels is akin to a magic cure? She rightly notes that "a strong, hardy, deep-seated depression will outsmart any chemical" [27] but also that "after an accumulation of life events made my head such an ugly thing to be stuck in, my brain's chemicals started to agree" [27]. Increased serotonin levels in the brain provide relief from a debilitating illness. Does it matter if the drug manufacturers are having a field day? "After all, what is depression if it isn't the most striking, poignant, psychic challenge to the American Dream" [27]?

Wurtzel has certainly had her detractors. It seems that overcoming one's life struggle can generate wariness and skepticism among those without a similar experience. Found among a collection of review snippets on Amazon.com: "Wurtzel is a very entertaining nut case..." says novelist Jeffrey Euginedes; In an issue of *Variety,* Todd McCarthy goes a step further in his review of the book's film: "The self-centered brat at the center of *Prozac Nation* spends most of her time making life miserable for everyone around her..." [29]. So, what to make of such statements?

Is describing one's suffering from such a mundane disease as depression a crime? Is this a kind of navel-gazing that uses self-pitying passages to glorify one's rank among the suffering [30]? Is it less to be debilitated by depression than to be afflicted by a brain tumor? One would think so based on such comments. However, a review in the *Library Journal* sheds more sympathetic tears: "Graphically written, this book expresses the pain and anger of Wurtzel's unremitting protest against her disability" [31]. And perhaps we can find balance in Michiko Kakutani's review in *The New York Times*:

> ...Ms. Wurtzel herself is hyperaware of the narcissistic nature of her problems, and her willingness to expose herself—narcissism and all—ultimately wins the reader over. By the end of "Prozac Nation," one is less apt to remember Ms. Wurtzel's self-important whining than her forthrightness, her humor and her ability to write sparkling, luminescent prose. [30]

It seems that Holly Ryan is right when she says, "Mental illness, specifically depression, has become so completely ubiquitous it seems fair game for satire" [32], which is unfortunate but perhaps a correlate to its very public success.

Prozac Diary

Eleven years following Prozac's introduction into the food chain in 1987, Penguin published Lauren Slater's *Prozac Diary*. She first started Prozac in 1988, taking it for the next ten years. Unlike *Prozac Nation,* in *Prozac Diary,* Slater spends more words getting at what Prozac does, how it makes you feel, and how it changes the way you see the world. There is less talk of illness and more of what seems like a cure. Slater does very well at entangling the reader in her depression, at showing us the dead ends of daily battle, and at giving us the profound relief she felt with Prozac.

Slater was very young when she first encountered a sadness that morphed into genuine depression. She says, "I think, yes, I was six or seven when I first felt it, the dwindling that is depression" [33]. Compare that to how she felt on Prozac in her twenties:

> This was what was different. It was as though I'd been vis-

ited by a blind piano tuner who had crept into my apartment at night, who had tweaked the ivory bones of my body, the taut strings in my skull, and now, when I pressed on myself, the same notes but with a mellower, fuller sound sprang out. [33]

Slater, though, sees through her bliss and does express misgivings regarding her recovery:

[B]ut life's become too good. Prozac's a drug you should take before you go on vacation, like to the Caribbean. They should sell this stuff in the CVS, along with Coppertone and beach thongs. I feel so damned relaxed. I can't really get anything creative done in this state. [33]

This mild damning of creativity is the subject of another chapter, but the writers in *Poets on Prozac* would disagree with Slater, saying that Prozac and medications like it make it possible to live, make it possible to be creative [34].

Artificial Happiness

Prozac has not only engendered glowing self-reports of efficacy and recovery, but has also reaped unprecedented scorn. Critics have biting words about the dangers of Prozac, specifically regarding its ability to change one's character, to alter one's being, as if that were a bad thing. It seems that one's authenticity is precious, even though a crippling disorder could be pushed to the side with treatment.

The very title of *Artificial Happiness: The Dark Side of the New Happy Class* by Ronald Dworkin (2006) names the assumed state of those taking antidepressants and promises to entertain with the "dark side" of this ill-begotten giddiness. According to Dworkin, "Artificial Happiness robs people...lifting them only halfway out of misery while preventing them from making the changes they need to make to enjoy real happiness" [35]. To be lifted out of misery, to someone who is merely depressed, though, is a very good thing. Right? There are certainly no changes coming while one is sniffing the dregs of one's soul laid bare to Churchill's black dog of depression.

This artificial happiness, "anchored in neurotransmitters and drugs," Dworkin equates with the pharmacogenic control of one's mind, body, and spirit [35], and physicians have roped this trinity with little pills. What does the patient have to say here? After all, it is their mind, body, and spirit. Eric Wilson claims, "My sense is that most of us have been duped by the American craze for happiness" [26], but what better to crave than happiness?

Whereas Wurtzel in *Prozac Nation* embraces her diagnosis and treatment, relishes in the vanquishing of her melancholy, Dworkin bemoans the happification of antidepressants, specifically the SSRIs such as Prozac. He thinks that "Doctors have taken on the responsibility of curing unhappiness... not depression... through artificial means" [35]. Dworkin says that people often need "a mass of unhappiness to push them out of a bad life situation" and that swallowing pills could delay a natural process of extricating oneself from the web of depression [35]. Dworkin spreads his net wide: "The medical profession now controls all three dimensions of life—the body, the mind, and the spirit—and clergymen have lost their relevance" [35]. And this is not a good thing according to Dworkin, seeming that doctors are worse than check forgers.

Dworkin sees this loss of self as unfortunate for the depressed, but gives doctors some license for their behavior, the presumed overprescribing of antidepressants, saying that "To the extent that they do mismanage patients, they do so unawares," rendering a class of patients he labels as "stupefied" [35]. Having attacked depression as an "engineering problem," Dworkin lapses hysterical, noting that "Through sheer numbers these people [doctors] pose a greater threat to the social fabric than murderers, prostitutes, and thieves" [35].

Perhaps less cantankerous than Dworkin, David Healy, in *Let Them Eat Prozac,* asserts that "depression was all but unrecognized before the antidepressants..." [36]. This is a chicken-and-egg scenario that devalues the lives of those who have always suffered more than mere sadness. Did people not commit suicide before the introduction of Prozac in 1987? One thing that Healy does for us is to trace the rise of antidepressants beginning with the introduction of the tricyclics (TCAs) and monoamine oxidase inhibitors (MAOIs) in 1957. As early as the 1960s, low serotonin levels were presented as a precursor to depression, possibly benefited by the early medications, but none more so than by the SSRIs to come. The first SSRI, zimelidine, was patented in 1972.

Let us return, though, to the dilemma of depression itself. How does depression make one feel? How desperate can one become to be relieved of the anguish? William Styron makes it clear that depression is insufferable. "[A] sense of self-hatred..." he calls it. "[A] general feeling of worthlessness...dark joylessness...a failure of self esteem..." [21]. Lying in bed with only thoughts of suicide, only thoughts of sheer despair, only a wicked darkness enveloping the soul, one would do most anything to escape. And it is this "ferocious inwardness of the pain" that propels one to grasp at straws, whether it be suicide or, better still, Prozac [21].

Elizabeth Wurtzel of *Prozac Nation* reminds us that "clinical depression...ruins lives..." [27]. Even the naysayer Charles Barber, the author of *Comfortably Numb: How Psychiatry Is Medicating a Nation,* says that "Many depressed people really, really want to die, and thinking about dying, or planning their death, takes up a great deal of time" [22].

Better than Well

Balancing this attack on Prozac and wellness stands a stalwart and highly reasonable researcher, psychiatrist Peter Kramer, the author of the classic *Listening to Prozac,* as well as *Against Depression,* and *Ordinarily Well,* which is a look back and defense of a decade of criticism leveled against *Listening to Prozac.* Kramer famously coined the term "cosmetic psychopharmacology," which has been taken by many as antidepressants being similar to a facelift. Kramer also coined the phrase "better than well" to describe some of his patients on Prozac and other antidepressants [37]. Is it okay to be better than well? Suppose you break your leg, receive a cast, heal, and then find you are a faster runner than before? Is there anything wrong with that? It seems that many, such as Glenmullen and Barber, are opposed to this "better than well" based on the assumption that it is not natural or that it bestows an unfair advantage. Who doesn't want to be "better than well," if indeed that is possible? Will we become like Goethe's Young Werther in one of his ecstasies: "A wonderful serenity has taken possession of my entire soul, like these sweet mornings of spring which I enjoy with my whole heart" [24]. Sounds pretty good.

But, to be fair, many are afraid of altering their psyche through medications, fearing they will not be themselves. "Some people...fear that psychoactive medications will change them..." [28]. Michael Norden notes, though, that "my patients who take Prozac...have never complained of any loss of identity" [28]. Still, the naysayers put loss of identity forward as inauthentic and worthy of shunning. Perhaps, like Young Werther, we fear our own gratification: "I treat my poor heart like a sick child, and gratify its every fancy" [24]. But what is one to do in the face of a disease that cripples? One seeks relief from the pain.

But still we worry. "It's all so neat and tidy," says Anna Moore. "There's something in you that is off balance and one little pill can right the wrong" [17]. In his article "The Silence of Prozac," K. Sharpe says, "Back then [1980s], I deeply resented 'having' to take the drugs, largely out of fear that they might change things about myself that I valued" [38]. But what about the things with hard value, such as the wrenching of one's soul, the inability to get out of bed, and missing days of productive life?

Even Glenmullen points us toward the known benefits of antidepressants. He says, "Certainly antidepressants can have an important place in a balanced, comprehensive psychiatric treatment. For patients with moderate to severe symptoms, judicious use of medication can be invaluable, even life-saving" [25]. But still we worry. Even Kramer says, "How much more uneasy will we be if doctors can reshape patients' social behavior in detail, through chemicals" [23]? He continues, noting that "We are justly suspicious of tonics for the normal brain" [23]. In a nod toward the naysayers, Kramer is honest: "[M]ood brighteners might decrease true autonomy by distancing man from an aspect of his humanity—his legitimate despair..." [23].

But, is this reaching normalcy an act of contrition? Do we all not desire to live a life free of those things that make us ill? Kramer notes that there are plenty of respected precedents for tackling what might be considered normal. He says, "The treatment of undesired nonpathologic conditions is common in medicine, such as estrogen to combat the normal effects of menopause" [23]. It is the idea of enhancement that is problematic. Menopause is a normal condition of life for older women, but is treating it an act of enhancement? Speaking of his father, Carl Elliott notes that

> Strictly speaking, 'enhancement' constituted a significant part of what my father, a small-town southern family doctor, has been doing in his office from the time he set up

shop in the late 1950s: immunizing children, freezing warts, removing moles and cysts. [39]

Are we to deprive children of immunizations simply because their lives are being enhanced?

James Edwards asks us about simple issues such as straighter teeth or clearer skin, which many seek. "How can we, who have (some) of these advantages—advantages in the games we indeed play—moralize carelessly about the others who want them" [40]? David DeGrazia points out a genuine humanitarian issue. He says that "One concern is that Prozac, and other pharmaceuticals that could be used for enhancement purposes, are not available to all who might want and stand to benefit from them" [41]. Is this not an argument for applying antidepressant technology to a wider audience? Worldwide, depression is the number one cause of disability [1]. Should we not be madly chasing down solutions, including humanitarian interventions, as we do with cancer and cardiovascular disease? As Laurence Kirmayer says, "There is a global monoculture of happiness in which we are all enjoined to work to achieve the good life..." [42]. And that is a good thing.

But the naysayers would differentiate between enhancement and authenticity. Elliot says, "The question is not just where there is any moral cost to the quest to become better, but whether there is any moral cost to the quest to become different" [39]. He wants the individual to look within for authenticity rather than taking medication. He even goes so far as to say that "The ideal of authenticity says that if you are not living a life as yourself, you have missed out on what life has to offer" [39]. But what if you are depressed and kill yourself? Is that authentic? Would it not have been better to seek treatment and live a full life in the shadow of a drug such as Prozac?

Wilson compares Prozac to "the two-beer buzz of canned

bliss" [26]. That is a bit reductionist, considering that wellness—a feeling of contentment with life—is something we all strive for. We all want straighter teeth. We all want to look forward to the next day. Is it the idea that, as part of a competitive society, those who take Prozac are somehow cheating and gaining an unfair advantage? Kramer asks, how might a drug "that alters personality...be used in a competitive society" [23]? That is a good question, but does competition not inherently imply a struggle to be the best? Someone who is depressed, who takes Prozac, may indeed acquire that "two-beer buzz," but they can do the same with beer. Should we discourage beer for fear that others may feel better than we do? How does a beer buzz foster inauthenticity? Does it matter that almost 85 percent of Americans already claim to be happy? [26]. Should we not root for the 15 percent who are not happy? Are they dangerous, a threat to our own happiness?

Sadness is a recurring theme among the critics of Prozac, who see in sadness a glorification of the human condition. Wilson says "...this quest for happiness at the expense of sadness, this obsession with joy without tumult, is dangerous, a deeply troubling loss of the real, of that interplay, rich and terrific, between antagonisms" [26]. But sadness does not simply cease to exist because one takes Prozac. The uplifting effect is not primal or all-encompassing. Life, sometimes a tough life, goes on regardless of medications taken, and it is very common for someone on an antidepressant to feel sad and even very depressed on a rougher day.

Prozac does not cure depression, but merely assuages its ragged corners, making life bearable. But still, "Enduring the sad existence is participating in life's vital rhythms" [26]. I would say that enduring a sad existence is not noble and that life's vital rhythms remain the same whether on or off Prozac. But Wilson hammers away: "Sadness reconciles us to realities. It throws us into the flow of life" [26]. If that is the case, then those among us who suffer from severe depression are riding class-six rapids and holding on for dear life. There is nothing wrong with a life jacket, whether the ship is sinking or not. Wilson continues, though, with this bit of philosophical whimsy: "Feeling totally alone, I experience union with all of the living. Suffering inevitable anxiety, I undergo a vital shock. I get it: to be alive is to realize the universe's grand polarity" [26]. Sounds romantic. But feeling totally alone without hope in the midst of a depressive episode is a terrible place to be, especially if self-harm rears its ugly head.

Wilson backs up his claims of sadness as life's spice with a quote from *Moby Dick:* "So, therefore, that mortal man who hath more of joy than sorrow in him, that mortal man cannot be true—not true, or undeveloped" [26]. Ahab was one man, and not a very happy man at that, being obsessed with the white whale. One can justify one's sad existence in any number of ways, including stigmatizing those who are not like us. But, again, those treated with Prozac do not necessarily have more joy than sorrow. The multifarious genetic and environmental components of depression create a substrate, a basic level of being that is capable of being lifted but not banished. Often, the term "crutch" is used for Prozac, but when we think of a man with a broken leg, the crutch makes perfect sense.

Is it the Prozac alone that is contributing to this supposed robbing of sadness, this dent to authenticity? Kramer says, "It is not only medicine that maintains well-being. Once we function competently, the world may pitch in" [23]. This is very true. Putting oneself on track brings oneself back to the world of the living. Spouses, children, and co-workers will take note of the change and "pitch in," as Kramer says. Why remain in a depressed and unproductive state when so many around us are counting on us? Is this pitching in of others then a blow to authenticity? No, it is called compassion. Some may call it self-interest. But, whatever it is called, the more help and support one receives while enduring a debilitating illness, the better. Kramer even notes that "For those who begin free of depression, antidepressants prove protective" [23]. This notion really raises the hackles of the naysayers and hints at the strong notion of being unfair. We want to prevent cancer, so why not depression?

Erik Parens, in a critique of Kramer's views, says that "Kramer goes to great pains to suggest that we—and he—need not be anxious about what Prozac will teach us regarding the authenticity of persons in general" [43]. As a clinical psychiatrist, we would expect that Kramer has the experience and knowledge to push aside authenticity as a panacea. He sees the proof in his patients on a daily basis. Discussing a patient of Kramer's profiled in *Listening to Prozac,* Parens notes that "Tess learned the authentic contours of her 'authentic self' from the drug" [43]. What is wrong with that? Has Tess obtained an unfair advantage by learning who her true self is? Rid of the chains of depression, has she evolved into some kind of super-human we must fear? Perhaps we can go as far as Elliott and Chambers to say that she has allowed herself to be boxed, but thus enabled to live [44]. If one has cancer, one is a victim of cancer. But it seems that if one has depression, then one is simply in a hole and relegated to stay there. Edwards notes that "The Tess that she had been on Prozac now seemed to her the true Tess" [40]. What is to fear of the true medicated self?

Parens whittles away at Kramer's notion of cosmetic psychopharmacology. He says that "...the more we use Prozac to build up our resistance to slights, the more we can expect such slights to proliferate" [43]. Is that logical? Will the world change because of those who claim treatment for sadness or depression? Parens indeed sees this as "morally problematic," but is it morally problematic to discover a case of high blood pressure and refuse to treat it? What to make of Parens' maxim that "Though one can find the self, one cannot actively change it..." [43]. Is the world not riddled with those who have overcome or perhaps degenerated into a different self? But he then says, "I believe such self-transformation can be quite admirable" [43]. One can change the basic self, if desired, but Prozac does not guarantee that as an outcome. Prozac merely treats the symptoms of depression, based on the theory that depressives suffer from a lack of certain neurotransmitters in the brain. It is not a matter of creating a Frankenstein, but of seeking a better self, not necessarily a new one.

One final quote from Parens: "[C]osmetic psychopharmacology can encourage social quietism" [43]. How does one prove this? Does taking Prozac create socially addled individuals incapable of processing information as "normal" people do? Is it not simply the desire to be "normal" that is the goal? If that is the case, then "already-normal" people should be subject to the same rules of social quietism.

Kramer, who has generated much of the criticism concerning Prozac, says that "my impression is that the concern over Prozac... turns almost entirely on an aesthetic valuation of melancholy" [45]. This is true. There seems to be a special place in the heart for sadness and the benefits it brings. One values the alcoholic writer who spends half of her time lying drunk in the gutter. Her writing is more real, more urgent. Would we value less the writings of Jack London, Sylvia Plath, or Virginia Woolf had they not killed themselves? Is the drowning of poet Paul Celan a cause for celebration of authenticity and trueness to self?

The True Self

Kramer has an interesting supposition here: "On a quest for authenticity, we must be open to discoveries of this sort—that what seemed to be a carefully developed self was arbitrary, biologically based idiosyncrasy" [45]. Genetics do play a role in depression, as does environment, just like most diseases that kill us. One's self develops as one ages, for better or for worse. Is this change in self a claim for disingenuity? "Is there a principled basis for linking melancholy to authenticity" [45]? That there is seems to be the staple of the naysayers' rhetoric, but there is little proof to support this claim. It just seems natural to assume that a medication alters one's self, whether for the better or the worse. But we need proof. And then we need to ask ourselves if it matters. Is an improved or different self better than living with depression, clutching at one's throat?

Some glorify the self as a natural condition untouched by pharmaceuticals. James Edwards says that "...when it comes to changing one's life (1) the natural way is better than the artificial, and (2) the hard way is better than the easy" [40]. Is it not difficult to admit to suffering from a stigmatizing disease and to seek help for it? Despite the surge in antidepressant prescriptions since the release of Prozac, suicide rates have not gone down. In 2015, suicide was the second leading cause of death among those aged 15 to 34. [46]. That is astounding. That is 12,438 lives that could have possibly been saved had the true self been sacrificed to something enhanced. And these are only the cases where suicide can be clearly proven. If Prozac can save a life, why all the attention to the concern over the true self?

Despite the damage caused by depression, there remains the adage of being obligated to pull oneself up by the bootstraps and muddle along as best one can. Says Edwards: "To be well is to exercise a particular sort of self-generated and well-ordered self-determination" [40]. That's well and good, but what resources do we have to facilitate that, and why is it suspect to use them? We live in an often-cruel world. We, the depressives, need a little help here. Elliot says,

> At least part of the nagging worry about Prozac and its ilk is that for all the good they do, the ills that they treat are part and parcel of the lonely, forgetful, and often unbearably sad place where we live. [47]

Yes, it is an unbearably sad place we live in, but hope exists.

We have the office worker in suburban America who no longer has the breath to leave his bed. Should we feel sorry for him? Should we just slap him on the back and say, "Giddyup?" Scholars, as Elliott says, may think that "Prozac treats the self rather than proper diseases" [47], but what is wrong with that if it makes life worth living? However, there is no category of disease called "self" in the *Diagnostic and Statistical Manual of Mental Disorders (DSM),* the Bible of psychiatric diagnosis, but there is quite a lengthy entry on depression, its symptoms and suggested treatment. If one wants science to uphold this idea of the self being a disease that can be treated, then we need research that supports that. If it takes the self as disease to help others, then let's make true self a disease.

Elliott asks, "When a person says, as did one man on Prozac, 'I don't have to look into the abyss anymore,' is he necessarily better off" [47]? Of course he is. It is not a matter of denying the abyss, but of being able to peek in and then look away, rather than fall in. We live in a stymied world. "Thus it is not happiness we seek, exactly, but the relief from the complexities of being" [48]. Ian Hacking quotes Richard Kluft: "Part of the socially prescribed role of being ill is working to recover and leave your illness behind" [49]. We want to feel better, to live. The abyss exists, more so for some than others, but it exists and is capable of sucking us down to oblivion. We desperately want to leave that behind.

Depression Since Prozac—Finding the True Self

There is that critique that Prozac and medications like it are created and marketed to generate illness, known as disease mongering. "Instead of creating drugs to treat diseases, we create diseases for which we can use our drugs" [7]. Is it true that "every society gets the doctors it deserves, and our doctors are merely giving us what we demand" [47]? We have cancer and we demand medications to cure it, to treat it, to alleviate suffering, and to prolong life. Arriving at the hospital in the throes of a heart attack, we expect the works. Why not the same with depression, the number one cause of disability worldwide?

Elliott makes authenticity a precursor to alienation, which he views as a good thing. This makes some say that "a person should be alienated—that given his or her circumstances, alienation is the proper response" [47]. However, Prozac will not take away that ability to feel alienated. By admitting to the disease, one experiences categorization and resultant alienation from those not affected. Being medicated is a form of alienation, although a welcome one. We all struggle to make sense of things, to understand our insignificance, and Prozac enables that sensibility.

Turning alienation toward psychic well-being, Elliott says this: "Here is the key to the problem psychiatry has with a notion like alienation. The measure of psychiatric success is internal psychic well-being...Whereas what I want to suggest is that maybe psychic well-being is not everything" [47]. Of course, one thing is not everything. But minimizing alienation and improving one's psychic well-being is a task that we all face. What if the measure of psychic well-being is simply staying alive to live a meaningful life? The depressed face this every day and deserve agents such as Prozac, even if it means becoming "better than well," much to the chagrin of Elliott and others.

Here is an interesting take on the issue of alienation and despair by Nasir Ghaemi: "A life without despair would be a life without hope, for hope cannot exist except as an antidote to despair" [7]. Ghaemi rightly examines the low points of life that enrich the high points. Locked away in a Birmingham jail, Martin Luther King Jr. rallied and wrote an impassioned plea and classic argument for an end to segregation. His turmoil, he turned to his advantage. But, in the grip of true depression, and not just mere sadness or perhaps rage, the vitality to rise to the occasion, which may simply be getting out of bed or writing a letter from jail, does not exist.

This brings us the broader issues surrounding alienation and despair. Says Hacking, "Love, passion, envy, tedium, regret, and quiet contentment are the stuff of the soul" [49]. Of course they are. Life is a smorgasbord of ups and downs. The plane is late, and we despair, but we have time to read a good book. We find ourselves in a rainstorm without an umbrella, and we take joy in splashing through the puddles. These are part of a life well lived, but free of crippling depression, which makes the late plane and the rain unbearable. How much better to be in a state of mind that is receptive to the simple mistakes of planes and clouds? Whether it is a two-beer buzz or Prozac, what does it matter?

Ghaemi, in his measured tone, asserts that "A little depression—not too much—makes you more realistic. No depression—none at all, being fully mentally healthy—makes you less realistic" [7]. Prozac may, on occasion, make you feel "better than well," but Prozac is not a cure for depression. Life's tribulations and the underlying disease go on. For the depressed and medicated, there will always remain that "little depression" and even bouts of severe depression that fight against all treatment given underlying genetic factors and environmental stressors. Prozac does not cure depression. There is no cure for depression, but thankfully, researchers are trying to get beyond this controversial notion of "better than well," which is transitory at best. In our toolbox, we have medications, psychotherapy, and even new experimental treatments such as the use of ketamine, which has shown great promise, equaling that of electroconvulsive therapy for the most serious of depression cases. It may be that "We experience pain so that we may live; without pain, we die" [7], but far too often it is that pain that ultimately leads to despair and possibly death by suicide or self-neglect.

Turning to the idea of sincerity as the measure of one's authenticity, whereby medications such as Prozac, according to Elliott, narrow "ordinary emotional range" [47], Lionel Trilling quotes Polonius from Shakespeare's Hamlet:

This above all: to thine own self be true
And doth it follow, as the night the day,
Thou canst not then be false to any man.

The naysayers would have us believe that being false, taking Prozac, renders one inauthentic, insincere. In the cunning sense of falsity, this may be true, but achieving well-being in the face of a debilitating disease is hardly cause to be labeled as false. Trilling helps to define this sincerity: "It derived from the Latin word sincerus and first meant exactly what the Latin words mean in its literal sense—clean, or sound, or pure...One spoke of sincere wine" [50]. How wonderful to be as sincere as a great wine, to be "clean, sound or pure." But it is the disease of depression that inhibits just that. Medications such as Prozac allow the wine to breathe and flower. Disease makes for bad wine.

Trilling, to emphasize his point, quotes a passage from "The Scarlet Letter": "Be true! Be True! Be true! Show freely to the world, if not your worst, yet some trait by which the worst may be inferred." Again, that message of authenticity that comes only from deep within the troubled soul. If anything, depressives must be the truest of us all, whether medicated or not. Depression does not mince words, and the worst may be inferred as suicide or a life hanging in the balance between utter despair and a groping for relief, whether it be pills or talk therapy. Goethe's Young Werther has this to say: "Human nature...has its limits. It is able to endure a certain degree of joy, sorrow, and pain, but becomes annihilated as soon as this measure is exceeded" [24].

Trilling explains why he holds this need to be true to oneself:

> Society requires of us that we present ourselves as being sincere, and the most efficacious way of satisfying this demand is to see to it that we really are sincere, that we are what we want our community to know we are. [50]

I think the key here is "to know who we are." To know and accept that one is depressed and in need of treatment is the first step toward this liberation. To take a drug such as Prozac and realize its benefits is a step toward revealing one's true potential, one's "true self." Without treatment, depression renders the individual helpless to meet society's demands that we really are sincere.

In the time that it has taken you to read this chapter, at least thirty sincere people worldwide have taken their lives. Although the rhetoric may seem cliché, that's one lethal act of authenticity every forty seconds [10].

What is Depression?

Depression, as Elizabeth Wurtzel says, "ruins...lives" [27]. But depression, as a widespread and popular term, only gained currency in the late 1980s, following the release of Prozac. According to David Healy,

> Depression as it is now understood by clinicians and at street level is therefore an extremely recent phenomenon, largely confined to the West. Its emergence coincides with the development of the selective serotonin reuptake inhibitors (SSRIs), [such as Prozac] which in the mid-1980s appeared capable of development as either anxiolytics or antidepressants. [51]

Prior to Prozac, released in 1987, the more generic term for depression, melancholia, was popular, a somewhat fluid and mysterious term that gives depression a notion of something otherworldly or even supernatural. *The Diagnostic and Statistical Manual of Mental Illness (DSM) V*, released in 2013, describes "Depressive Disorders," which includes major depressive disorder. According to Rebecca Clay, the *DSM-V*, "incorporates new findings while taking into account mental health professionals' need for consistency..." [52]. Clay, quoting Chris Hopwood, says that the latest version of the *DSM* is a move "toward more evidence-based models on the one hand and the need to not disrupt clinical practice as it stands..." [52]. The *DSM-IV*, released in 1994, gathered depression into "Mood Disorders," which includes major depressive disorder. The *DSM-III*, released in 1980, described "Affective Disorders," which included major depression. A great leap occurred from the *DSM-II* to the *DSM-III,* growing from 119 pages to 472 pages. The *DSM-II,* released in 1968, described "major affective disorders" as a subgroup of "psychoses not attributed to physical conditions listed previously." Within major affective disorders, depression in general was described as "involutional melancholia," with the term depression only occurring in conjunction with manic-depressive illness. The *DSM-I,* released in 1952, referenced "severe depression," but as a component of "Psychotic Disorders," such as schizophrenia. Depression was also listed as a "defense" against anxiety and as a component of chronic brain syndrome. The most direct reference to depression was as a "psychotic depressive reaction" [53]. Thus, at least since the advent of the *DSM* series in 1952, depression has been winding along a road from a symptom of madness to a bona fide diagnosis with specific treatments that can be verified by clinical research.

In coming to terms with depression as a diagnosis, there is now a tendency to see depression as a continuum, which is logical, ranging from sadness to severe depression. The key to diagnosis is when to recognize depression as an illness versus just a normal reaction to the harshness of life. Sadness, we have noted, is valued as part of a meaningful life. Revisiting a quote from Joseph Glenmullen, "Genuine sadness is quite different from depression. Sadness is a clarifying, relieving emotion that helps one move on after losses" [25]. So, accepting that, it is vitally important to know when that clarifying sadness leaks into true depression. If we take the WHO's stance that "health is a state of complete physical, mental and social well-being and not merely the absence of disease or infirmity," [54] we may want to consider that depression ranges into sadness and that treatment may be desirable even at that "lesser" state of depression. One does not have to be psychotic to be miserable and in need of relief [55].

Depression Since Prozac—Finding the True Self

According to historian Edward Shorter, psychiatry is a relatively new medical discipline. It wasn't until 1808 that Johann Christian Reil "coined the term psychiatry...for the new discipline" [18]. At that point in time, depression, if recognized at all, was deemed as a variety of insanity or demon possession and most often earned the term "melancholia," which falls short of a disease needing treatment. The "father" of American psychiatry, Benjamin Rush, published in 1812 his *Observations and Inquiries upon the Diseases of the Mind,* which took the progressive view that mental illness was a disease, an affliction of the mind. In 1852, the physician Heinrich Laehr noted that "insanity is nothing else than a disease, and only medical treatment can prevail against it" [18].

Back to the topic, "What is depression?" What is it about this "...ferocious inwardness of the pain..." [21] that calls for recognition as a legitimate concern for hundreds of millions of people worldwide? As a reminder, depression is the number one cause of disability worldwide, "and is a major contributor to the overall global burden of disease" [1]. Worldwide, more than 300 million people suffer from depression, which, at its worst, can lead to suicide [1]. The good news is that there are proven treatments, including therapy and medications such as Prozac. Michael Norden says, "A recent study found that surprisingly, the impairment associated with minor depression often exceeded that caused by medical conditions such as heart disease, diabetes, and arthritis" [28]. Depression, which develops from one's environmental circumstances and genetic makeup, is a complex beast with wide-ranging damage. Says Charles Barber, "Psychiatric disorders are almost certainly the dialectical product of an infinitely complex dialogue between genes and the environment" [22]. And we are reminded by Peter Kramer that "people don't have to be made vulnerable by trauma: they can be born vulnerable" [23].

Depression compromises the body and the soul. As Wurtzel says,

> The…depressed are more likely to be walking wounded, people like me who are quite functional, whose lives proceed almost as usual, except that they're depressed all the time, almost constantly embroiled in thoughts of suicide even as they go through their paces. [27]

Yes, the depressed do walk and talk, but often with a thick layer of lead that fosters thoughts of hopelessness and self-harm. And it is often the case that being diagnosed is a relief in itself. You have a name for what is dogging you. Wurtzel found this liberating. "I had fallen in love with my depression…I loved it because I thought it was all I had" [27]. Strange, but often true. Some might say, "Embrace your diagnosis. Let it work for you."

Turning briefly to examine how our language describes depression, Kimberly Emmons notes,

> The language of depression implicates both healthy and ill individuals, and it encourages particular orientations of the self and legitimizes patterns of gendered behavior that have physical and social ramifications. Depression is, therefore, a rhetorical illness; it functions persuasively in our collective and individual consciousness. [56]

This is interesting. Depression is a medical diagnosis, such as major depressive disorder, the details of which perhaps remain unknown to the average person. But they can grasp the word, the idea, the language, and apply that to those fitting the mold of the popular notion of depression. This is largely thanks to medications such as Prozac, which have opened the door to visualizing and becoming comfortable with depression as a common disorder. Although "Depression has become, according to one popular mental health website, 'the common cold of mental disorders'" [56]. But at least it is no longer associated with demons or as simply a symptom of something broader, such as schizophrenia. Depression is now a living thing, a thing with a face

Further, Emmons speaks of a "vocabulary of deficit" in relation to describing depression. She borrows this idea from Kenneth Gurgen. As an example, she provides us with a National Institute of Mental Health brochure that describes the depressed as "'lacking in zest and enthusiasm for life'" [56]. So, depression is the lack of something. It is a simple way to grasp a complex issue. Persons with AIDS lack functioning T-cells. Persons with Meniere's disease lack balance. Persons who wear glasses may lack good vision. This leaves us with a gap that needs to be filled. And what better to fill a gap than with proven treatments such as Prozac or cognitive behavioral therapy? Holly Ryan says, "In our day-to-day behaviors and interactions with others, certain codes of conduct are normal while others, especially sadness, loneliness, or apathy, are not" [32]. It is difficult not being able to read due to impaired vision, but it is okay. It is fixable, the same as with depression. Embracing your diagnosis takes that extra step to realize that you are not entirely normal, that something is wrong.

Ryan is critical of medications such as Prozac, though. He says, "Whereas in the past, people were expected to pull themselves up by their bootstraps or seek advice from friends, family, or priests, now medicine will do it for them" [32]. Thus, and this is a problem, depression that is "not too bad," that is merely "sadness," may be downplayed as a character flaw that, if treated with medications, indicates weakness, an inability to grab the bootstraps and yank. Barber says, "A study of antidepressant use in private health insurance plans found that a majority of those prescribed antidepressants received no psychiatric diagnosis or any mental health care beyond the prescription of the drug" [22]. Withholding a diagnosis for depression leaves the patient uncertain and without incentive to perhaps seek additional care, such as psychotherapy. Even with the increasing acceptance of depression as a disease worthy of treatment, many of the depressed still avoid the stigma of visiting a psychiatrist and rely on their family doctor for treatment. But, also, perhaps it is the case that the patient wants the medication but not the diagnosis.

Dan Blazer, author of *The Age of Melancholy*, has much to say about what depression is. He quotes Robert Burton: Depression is "a kind of dotage without fever, having for his ordinary companions fear and sadness, without any apparent occasion" [57]. This is an excellent description of depression, describing its symptoms as companions. Indeed, depression makes itself known upon waking and follows one throughout the day and into the night, and even into the dream life. It is this "loss of orientation, meaning, and hope" that defines daily life of the depressed, which day after day becomes unbearable without treatment [57]. Says Blazer, "Depression is at once body, mind, and environment. Depression is at once endogenous and exogenous" [57]. Depression is all-encompassing, all devastating, and represents a reaction to the stressors of life, along with biological dysfunction such as the lack of serotonin in the brain. Depression affects every aspect of life, including decisions both big and small. People lose their jobs because of depression. People kill themselves because of depression. Blazer notes, "Low mood might help people to disengage from pursuing a goal that is perceived to be unattainable" [57]. One cannot move forward while depressed and simply tries to hold on to each painful moment, wishing the despair away.

Although Wilson says, "We are right now at this moment annihilating melancholia" [26], Peter Kramer notes that depression is "a progressive, probably lifelong disorder" [23]. Says Norden,

> For people who have had two or three previous episodes of major depression, psychiatrists now often recommend indefinite treatment to foil the high odds of recurrence. After three episodes of depression, recurrence runs about 90 percent... [28]

Some people are born with the tendency toward depression. Others develop depression in response to a life event such as a death or divorce. Kramer notes that "psychosocial stressors like pain, isolation, confinement, and lack of control can lead to structural changes in the brain and can kindle progressively more autonomous acute symptoms" [23]. Just as diabetes causes permanent damage, such as the destruction of small blood vessels in the extremities, depression accumulates like plaque in an artery, altering one's physical condition as the disease progresses. Kramer is wary of those clinicians who are reluctant to treat depression with medications such as Prozac. Is it right to discover a case of depression and withhold treatment? Kramer is optimistic, though: "It is at least possible that we will someday advocate early detection of depression the way we now advocate early detection of cancer or hypertension, and that treatment of nearly normal conditions will become standard preventive medicine" [23].

Describing depression, Kramer says, "Among the most enduring traits of depressive personality are introversion and social maladroitness..." [23]. There are those who are shy and awkward and not depressed, but that inability to press forward out of fear engendered by depression can be a very real stumbling block to one's satisfaction with life. Concerning depression and authenticity, discussed earlier, the depressed still have to battle for their basic right to happiness. Says Wilson,

> I for one am afraid that our American culture's overemphasis on happiness at the expense of sadness might be dangerous, a wanton forgetting of an essential part of a full life" [26]. But what about that painful inability to look another in the eye and speak with confidence? Depression debilitates, robbing one of happiness and confidence. Untreated depression is never part of a 'full life.' [26]

Is there an upside to depression? Quoting Thomas Sydenham, Michel Foucault notes that "melancholics 'are people, who, apart from their complaint, are prudent and sensible, and who have an extraordinary penetration and sagacity.' Thus Aristotle rightly observed that melancholics have more intelligence than other men" [58]. The key here is to reach out and link these positive traits with a disorder such as depression. Depressives often do dig down deep and force themselves upon the world, earning admiration for their prudence and sensibility. There is a connection with the pain of life that can bring lasting insights into empathy and goodwill, but ultimately these kind traits are erased by incessant self-loathing and, often, a desire to just end it all. Treating the depressed, contrary to Wilson, though, will not rob the depressed of their ability to wage goodwill, but will only strengthen it. Foucault says, "For when melancholia fixes upon an aberrant idea, it is not only the soul which is involved; it is the soul within the brain..." [58]. Foucault is right. Depression, melancholia, is a disorder of the brain and of the very soul, which will cry out for help when one's defensive mechanisms are exhausted.

The "oppression of the soul" experienced by a group of women in Ethiopia [6] is apt whether you are the survivor of a famine or a bedraggled office worker. Laurence Kirmayer has examined depression in Japan and has some interesting insights.

> In Japan, depression has wide recognition as a notion, but there is no exact translation of the English word. Japanese terms usually glossed in English as 'melancholy' or 'depression' include yuutsu (related to grief but also to gloominess of spirits and weather); ki ga meiru (ki is leaky); shizumu (low in spirits)... [42]

So, there is depression across cultures, loudly seconded by the WHO and the *World Happiness Report,* but it may be called by different names. The sorrow of one's soul, the lack of serotonin, the drudgery of life, and the inability to face the day are ubiquitous throughout the world. A depressive in Canada will recognize the same in Zimbabwe. Kirmayer brings our attention to an interesting Japanese word: ikigai, which translates as "that which makes one's life seem worth living" [42]. It is this ikigai, this universal right not to be depressed, that is all important, and we have the medications and science to facilitate just that. It is important to remember that "While one in five Americans lives with a mental health condition, only about 50 percent of those people receive mental health services" [19]. Let's find them and give them relief.

Observing Elizabeth Wurtzel and her enthusiastic embrace of her diagnosis as a means to an end, Wilson hesitates, saying, "I don't want to romanticize clinical depression" [26]. He continues, as mentioned earlier, "My sense is that most of us have been duped by the American craze for happiness" [26]. No one has been duped unless they have not had the opportunity for relief. If there should ever be a craze, it should be for happiness. What better cause could there be? Depressives precisely lack this happiness, which is a basic human right. Whether cocooned within riches or a burger flipper, we deserve the ability to see clearly and not to be blinded by an ubiquitous illness that responds so very well to a variety of treatments, including Prozac and medications like it. Wilson detours a bit, bringing us to the *Declaration of Independence:*

> In this document, of course, we learn that everyone enjoys an inalienable right to 'life, liberty, and the pursuit of happiness.' What many of us don't know, though, is that 'the pursuit of happiness' is secretly connected to the ownership of property...the true road to earthly joy is through the accumulation of stuff. [26]

Perhaps he is not truly serious? Often, to a depressive, happiness is merely opening one's eyes in the morning and not thinking of death, versus owning twenty acres in the country.

Foucault, in his classic, *Madness and Civilization,* lumps all mental illness into "madness," which is problematic and archaic, but there is a point when depression is so ugly that one truly feels crazed or mad. The benefit of saying "madness" is that it gives Foucault license to speak broadly of the disorders that afflict the mind. He says, "Madness begins where the relation of man to truth is disturbed and darkened" [58]. That's another great insight into the disease of depression. Perhaps his best summary of depression, and madness, is that one suffers from one's "reason [being] dazzled" [58]. This plays well into Kramer's "introversion and social maladroitness" as traits of depression [23]. One is dazzled into oblivion. One often does not recognize the insidiousness of depression, and often it is the job of loved ones to guide the depressive toward treatment lest they become completely disabled.

For "madness" as a sum of mental illness, Foucault has this somewhat brutal observation, which highlights the physical aggression of depression and other disorders:

Depression Since Prozac—Finding the True Self

It is this languishing flow, these choked vessels, this heavy, clogged blood that the heart labors to distribute throughout the organism, and which has difficulty penetrating in the very fine arterioles of the brain, where the circulation ought to be very rapid in order to maintain the movement of thought—it is all this distressing obstruction which explains melancholia...The explanation becomes a transfer to the organism of qualities perceived in the condition, the conduct, the words of the sick person. We move from qualitative apprehension to supposed explanation. But it is this apprehension that continues to prevail and always wins out over theoretical coherence. [58]

As with Foucault, and as shown in the evolution of the APA's *DSM* series, there is a strong desire to make some theoretical coherence out of mental illness. We want evidence. We want to be able to definitively diagnose depression and then apply proven treatments that battle the recognized traits of the disorder. We want a cure, just as we do with cancer. But like cancer, there is as yet no cure for depression, only treatments that render it less deadly. Says Kramer, speaking of a milder form of depression, dysthymia: "Dysthymia is debilitating. Studies show that in the long run, endless minor symptoms are as disabling as severe episodes spaced out in time" [23]. Listening to Foucault, the vessels are choked, the heart heavy with clogged blood. More clinically exact than Foucault, Herman van Praag says, "Depression is a syndrome composed of a multitude of psychopathological dimensions, of which mood-lowering is generally considered to be the major one" [59]. Although more practical, van Praag's view of depression lacks the drama of Foucault, which better gets at the destruction of the soul that depression brings.

Depression is a disease, one that is well classified and examined in the *DSM-V*. Nasir Ghaemi would qualify this, though:

It has become de rigueur to state that depression is a disease. The part of it that is recurrent and episodic, or due to a specific medical cause, is disease. But the part that is not episodic, but that is chronic and admixed with anxiety, becomes indistinguishable from personality... [7]

But, whether or not depression is part of one's personality, and it will become a part of one's identity whether wanted or not, depression "ruins...lives" [27]. As Goethe's Young Werther so poignantly states, "The leaven which animated my existence is gone: the charm which cheered me in the gloom of night, and aroused me from my morning slumbers, is for ever fled" [24].

The Severity and Spread of Depression

Depression is the number one cause of disability worldwide and affects more than 300 million people [1]. Depression alone is a disease that slows, cripples, and kills. Depression also worsens other conditions, such as heart disease and other mental illnesses, such as anxiety disorders and eating disorders [3]. According to the CDC, More than 1 out of 20 Americans 12 years of age and older reported current depression between 2009 and 2012 [3]. According to the National Institute of Mental Health, an estimated 16.1 million adults aged 18 or older in the United States had at least one major depressive episode in the past year (2014), representing 6.7 percent of all U.S. adults [4]. Further, as noted previously, "In a given year, almost a third of American adults with major depression receive no medical attention for it" [23]. These statistics highlight the need for intensive interventions to treat those afflicted and to bring relief to those not currently treated.

According to Anna Moore, "Studies suggest that in America, depression more than doubled between 1991 and 2001" [17]. This was a period of time in which more medications like Prozac were being released and championed. A public discourse on depression was in full swing, set into motion by Wurtzel's *Prozac Nation* with a concurrent flood of research studies on the pros and cons of the new class of antidepressant medications that targeted neurotransmitters such as serotonin and norepinephrine. Depression had come out of the closet. It was now firmly named and classified as a unique disease that responds well to treatment. The rise in depression rates can thus be attributed to people being more willing to seek treatment, to seek the new medications to treat depression, and to doctors being more aware and better able to diagnose and treat depression.

One way to view this doubling of depression numbers is to look at the prescriptions of antidepressants. To visualize the jump in prescription rates of antidepressants from 1988 through 2012, the CDC has gathered data that describes the percentage of the population that has been prescribed an antidepressant in the last 30 days. Across all age groups, the percentage climbs proportionally across the years. The percentage for those 18 to 44 years jumped from 1.6 percent (1988-1994) to 8.4 percent (2009-2012), an increase of 352 percent. The increases are similar for those in the 45-to-over-75 age groups [20]. One can surmise that as new treatments became available, such as Prozac in 1987, and as the public became more aware and more comfortable with recognizing depression as a legitimate illness, that antidepressant interventions became more prevalent and popular. Critics such as Healy refer to this as disease mongering [7]. But, of course, depression is not a disease that has to be created. It has always existed, whether called madness, melancholia, or major depressive disorder. Since the release and discussion of Prozac and depression, it has simply become more acceptable to prescribe antidepressants, as well as easier to diagnose. The parameters for diagnosing depression have become more honed and reliable based on empirical evidence. Antidepressants such as Prozac work very well and deserve the attention, both positive and negative, they have received.

The CDC has also measured the population percentage of severe psychological distress from 1997 through 2013. Overall, the rate has remained relatively stable, fluctuating from a low of 2.6 percent to a high of 3.4 percent, representing a percentage change of 31 percent [60]. This indicates that the increase in antidepressant prescriptions is not closely linked with serious psychological distress but is associated with minor to moderate psychological distress. This puts more pressure on the increase in antidepressant prescriptions to reveal that there is a corresponding need for those prescriptions. But perhaps the rates of distress would be much higher were medications such as Prozac not available. Again, are doctors prescribing more and more antidepressants simply because they can, or is there a genuine medical need? As always, more study is needed, but the assumption that perhaps physicians are looking harder for depression may explain the vast increase in antidepressant prescriptions, which is a good thing for those who need it.

In 1980, seven years prior to Prozac, a study using a self-report questionnaire showed "that primary physicians failed to diagnose about 50 percent of both depressed and otherwise impaired patients" [61]. The results were obtained by comparing a review of medical charts for the diagnosis of depression with the results of the questionnaire known as the Beck Depression Inventory (BDI). Using the BDI scores, A.C. Nielsen and T.A. Williams arrived at a 12.2 percent prevalence of depression when "mild depression was used as a criterion" [61]. Moderate depression rated at 5.5 percent, while severe depression described 0.6 percent of the population [61]. It appears that the BDI is a better screening tool than the primary physician, but as time has passed, primary care physicians have become more aware of tests such as the BDI and are more willing to use them. This is an important consideration, especially since many patients were undiagnosed and without treatment. Also, in addition to possibly saving lives and making lives more bearable, "the identification and treatment of psychiatric problems in medical populations has been shown to diminish the use and overall costs of medical services in prepaid medical plans" [61]. This suggests that there is a correlation between diseases such as depression and one's overall physical health.

The Cost of Depression

Depression is expensive and affects 300 million people worldwide. There are the obvious costs, such as those for treatment, but what about the social costs and the additional costs that depression adds to other diseases? How many sick days are wasted on depression? How many job opportunities are missed because one can't get out of bed? Those are tough things to measure. But there is data that allows us to examine the financial burden of depression.

In total, American healthcare costs by 2013 amounted to $2.92 trillion dollars. This means that, based on a population of 320 million people in the US, the average cost per person was about $9,200. This amount is projected to increase to $4.3 trillion by 2020, averaging $12,741 per person [62]. In 1980, the total economic cost of illness was estimated at $455 billion. Of that, 6.7 percent, or $30.7 billion, was attributed to mental disorders [63]. In looking at depression costs from 1990 to 2000, P.E. Greenberg et al. found that even though depression diagnoses increased over 50 percent, "its economic burden rose by only 7 percent, going from 77.4 billion dollars in 1990 (inflation-adjusted dollars) to 83.1 billion dollars in 2000" [64]. Jumping to 2010, according to the CDC, "The economic burden of depression, including workplace costs, direct costs and suicide-related costs, was estimated to be $210.5

billion in 2010" [3]. How much of this cost is related to increased awareness of depression is hard to say, but it must play a role. Much of the cost is also hidden. According to the American Psychological Association, "For every dollar spent on MDD [major depressive disorder] direct costs in 2010, an additional $1.90 was spent on MDD-related indirect costs..." [65]. The largest portion, of course, is direct medical costs, which include prescription medications such as Prozac. According to Ghaemi,

> ...psychiatric medicines are second only to cardiology drugs as the most profit-making class of drugs in the world..." [7]. However, "Effective treatment of depression with fluoxetine [Prozac] and other SSRIs not only reduces the suffering and disability of patients, but decreases the cost of healthcare owing to the reoccurrence of depression. [66]

Comparing health claims costs of workers with depression to those without depression, Blazer found that

> [I]n one study of more than 15,000 employees of a major U.S. corporation that filed health claims in 1995, workers with depression incurred an average of $1,341 in mental health care costs and $3,032 in nonmental health care, more total than workers with diabetes, heart disease, and depression...That translated into $2.2 million total expenses to the corporation secondary to depression. [57]

Treating depression can be expensive, but it must be compared to the costs of not treating it. Suicide alone costs society over $44.6 billion a year in combined medical and work loss costs [9]. Each suicide, factoring in lost wages of the deceased, costs society $1,164,499 [9].

Depression Since Prozac—Finding the True Self

The costs of depression, other than treatment, include many socioeconomic factors that may be taken for granted. According to Ronald Kessler, these include:

> low educational attainment, high risk of teen childbearing, marital disruption, and unstable employment. Among people with specific social and productive roles, MDD [major depressive disorder] is found to predict significant decrements in role functioning (e.g., low marital quality, low work performance, low earnings). MDD is also associated with elevated risk of onset, persistence, and severity of a wide range of chronic physical disorders as well as with increased early mortality due to an even wider range of physical disorders and to suicide. [67]

And these disruptions in one's ability to earn and contribute are chronic. Kessler says, "clinical studies show that a substantial proportion of people who seek treatment for major depression have a chronic-recurrent course of illness" [67]. Thus, depression can be seen as a lifelong illness that accumulates costs year after year, especially when left untreated. "One of the most striking aspects of the impairment associated with MDD is that the personal earnings and household income of people with MDD are substantially lower than those of people without depression" [67]. Major depressive disorder, according to Kessler, is associated with a wide variety of illnesses, including "arthritis, asthma, cancer, cardiovascular disease, diabetes, hypertension, chronic respiratory disorders, and a variety of chronic pain conditions," and the costs of these conditions can be factored as costs of depression [67]. Thus, the costs of depression are wide-ranging, and treatment could reduce costs of illnesses that are comorbid with depression. According to Martin Knapp, "The effect of depression on employment (and hence on national productivity) in cost terms is 23 times larger than the costs falling to the health service" [68]. He refers to this as a hidden cost, but one that is very real. According to P.E. Greenberg et al. (2015), the costs of MDD can be broken down as follows: "approximately 45 percent attributable to direct costs, 5 percent to suicide-related costs, and 50 percent to workplace costs. Only 38 percent of the total costs were due to MDD itself as opposed to comorbid conditions" [69]. The costs of depression are many, which can often be summed up not only by monetary costs but also by Wurtzel's notion of ruined lives [27].

Given that healthcare costs are expected to rise by 6.5 percent in 2018 [70], healthcare providers will seek ways to cut costs and reduce utilization. As there are already so many who are without treatment for mental disorders such as depression, we need to remember the hidden costs of depression and attack the disease head-on with professional treatment that keeps these hidden costs in mind. It can be surmised that it is more expensive to not treat depression than it is to treat depression. The Affordable Care Act (ACA), signed into law in 2010, became fully effective in 2014 and insured an additional 24 million people in 2016 alone. According to the CDC, "The percentage of persons uninsured... decreased, from 16.0 percent in 2010 to 8.9 percent in January–June 2016" [71], roughly 224,000 persons newly insured. Without the ACA, many with mental illnesses, such as depression, and newly able to afford treatment, will find themselves once again alone in their battle for sanity. According to *The Washington Post*, "Repealing the Affordable Care Act will kill more than 43,000 people annually" [72].

On a final note, the wrath of costs attributed to diseases such as depression is often foisted on the medical establishment and pharmaceutical companies in general. According to Ghaemi, referencing postmodernism,

One symptom of postmodernism is the attack on the motivations of others. Commonly, motivations are presumed to be financial: everything is about money; hence postmodernists go on the warpath against the pharmaceutical industry and its collaborators in academic medicine. [7]

Of course, the establishment wants to make money, but they are making viable and effective treatment options available to those who are lucky enough to receive them. Greed may be a symptom of our times, but that is nothing new. What is new since the release of Prozac is the public's and the establishment's recognition that depression exists and that it deserves the same careful attention as any other major disorder, such as cancer or heart disease.

Are We Happy Yet?

Another way to recognize depression is by looking at happiness. In 2006, the Pew Research Center conducted a happiness survey for the United States, using a telephone interview of a nationally representative, randomly-selected sample of 3,014 adults:

> Just a third (34 percent) of adults in this country say they're very happy, according to the latest Pew Research Center survey. Another half say they are pretty happy and 15 percent consider themselves not too happy. These numbers have remained very stable for a very long time. [2]

Although this unhappiness is not equal to depression, which has a variety of defined symptoms, according to the APA's *DSM-V*, it gives us an idea of one of the major symptoms of depression, happiness. The 15 percent who are "not too happy" roughly correlates with the 12.2 percent prevalence of depression described by Nielsen and Williams, which includes those with mild depression.

Income can be one major player in whether or not one is happy.

> Our survey shows that nearly half (49 percent) of those with an annual family income of more than $100,000 say they're very happy. By contrast, just 24 percent of those with an annual family income of less than $30,000 say they're very happy. [2]

Life events and the environment are also a contributor to unhappiness and depression.

> Much of the research into the field of happiness—to say nothing of simple common sense—suggests that at the level of the individual, happiness is heavily influenced by life events (Did you get the big promotion? Have a fight with your boyfriend?) as well as by psychological traits (self-esteem, optimism, a sense of belonging, the capacity to love, etc.). [2]

And so, we have "common sense" as an indicator of happiness as well as "psychological traits," which, since the release of Prozac, have become more ubiquitous in diagnosing depression. We have, by 2006, the year of the Pew study, and six years after the release of Prozac, a solid footing in the diagnosis and treatment of unhappiness and depression, which formerly existed solely in the pages of the *DSM* and doctors' offices and not in the popular mind.

Here are more findings from the Pew study:

> Married people are happier than unmarrieds. People who worship frequently are happier than those who don't. Republicans are happier than Democrats. Rich people are

happier than poor people. Whites and Hispanics are happier than Blacks. Sunbelt residents are happier than those who live in the rest of the country. We also found some interesting non-correlations. People who have children are no happier than those who don't, after controlling for marital status. Retirees are no happier than workers. Pet owners are no happier than those without pets. [2]

Here we have a somewhat rounded view of what it is like to be happy. You are more likely to be happy if you are wealthy, married, a Republican, white or Hispanic, and live in a sunbelt state. But then there are the 15 percent who are unhappy and the 12.2 percent who are diagnosed with depression, and it very well may be that you are wealthy or married but still depressed.

The Pew report continues: "Here most of the findings are pretty predictable—healthier people tend to be happier, and so do better-educated people" [2]. It seems, as common sense says, that if you are healthy, then you are more likely to be happy. One's good health is the greatest gift that one has. But if you are depressed, then you are not healthy. And if you suffer from cardiac disease, then you may be more likely to develop depression as a response, compounding the disease. However, depression may also be linked to developing cardiac and other diseases, resulting in that same compounding of illness. According to D.L. Hare et al.,

> Patients with CVD [cardiovascular disease] have more depression than the general population. Persons with depression are more likely to eventually develop CVD and also have a higher mortality rate than the general population. Patients with CVD, who are also depressed, have a worse outcome than those patients who are not depressed. There is a graded relationship: the more severe the depres-

sion, the higher the subsequent risk of mortality and other cardiovascular events. [73]

The Pew survey sums up its findings by saying, "Even so, the factor that makes the most difference in predicting happiness is neither being a Republican nor being wealthy—it is being in good health" [2]. And treating depression, whether it be Prozac or psychotherapy, or both, is what is needed for good health. Not only does treating depression increase happiness and well-being, but it also possibly reduces the severity of other diseases and decreases overall health costs [61].

An interesting additional factor to one's happiness is whether or not one is a parent. According to John Helliwell, Richard Layard, and Jeffrey Sachs,

> Looking across the world, a negative relationship between parenthood and life satisfaction is found in two-thirds of the countries studied. The negative effect of parenthood on life satisfaction is found to be significantly stronger in countries with higher GDP per capita or higher unemployment rates. [74]

Thus, whether or not one is happy is very complicated. For example, having children is stressful physically, mentally, and financially. The takeaway is that those who are depressed are a colorful variety of people, many of whom you would expect to be depressed, but some who you would not expect to be depressed. For many, depression begins with one's genetic makeup. You are destined to be prone to depression [75] and deserve watching. Scientists have even discovered a specific gene located at chromosome 3p25-26 that seems to influence depression [76].

The *World Happiness Report*

This happiness or unhappiness in the United States is further addressed by the World Happiness Report, in its fifth edition, first published in 2012 as part of the High Level Meeting at the United Nations on Happiness and Well-Being [74]. The report covers more than 150 countries, with 1,000 individual life evaluations taken in each country. The basic method is this question:

> Please imagine a ladder, with steps numbered from 0 at the bottom to 10 at the top. The top of the ladder represents the best possible life for you and the bottom of the ladder represents the worst possible life for you. On which step of the ladder would you say you personally feel you stand at this time? [74]

Thus, this is an elementary study, but one that yields consistent results. Six key variables determine the differences in the scores of each country:

> The six factors are GDP per capita, healthy years of life expectancy, social support (as measured by having someone to count on in times of trouble), trust (as measured by a perceived absence of corruption in government and business), perceived freedom to make life decisions, and generosity (as measured by recent donations). Differences in social support, incomes and healthy life expectancy are the three most important factors. [74]

These variables again ring of common sense and point to the role of feeling secure and being healthy as keys to happiness. Whether living in a refugee camp in Sudan or toiling in a Portland cubicle, people around the world need to feel some control over their destiny and overall health, measured here by social support, income, and life expectancy. According to the report:

> The cause of happiness as a primary goal for public policy continues to make good progress. So far, four national governments—Bhutan, Ecuador, United Arab Emirates and Venezuela—have appointed ministers of happiness responsible for coordinating their national efforts. [74]

That is far-reaching and far-sighted on behalf of those countries, even if they are interested only in productivity. Even companies have jumped on the bandwagon, appointing directors of happiness to boost morale, reward employees, and increase productivity. One such company is Lamp Post Group in Chattanooga, Tennessee, a venture incubator that provides both capital and mentorship to growing startups. One recruiting website (indeed.com), in 2017, listed 1,137 jobs related to guiding employee happiness and well-being.

Here are the latest top ten happiest and bottom ten happiest countries surveyed by the *World Happiness Report*:

Top 10 happiest countries:
1. Denmark (7.526)
2. Switzerland (7.509)
3. Iceland (7.501)
4. Norway (7.498)
5. Finland (7.413)
6. Canada (7.404)
7. Netherlands (7.339)
8. New Zealand (7.334)
9. Australia (7.313)
10. Sweden (7.291)

Bottom ten happiest countries:
148. Madagascar (3.695)
149. Tanzania (3.666)
150. Liberia (3.622)
151. Guinea (3.607)
152. Rwanda (3.515)
153. Benin (3.484)
154. Afghanistan (3.360)
155. Togo (3.303)
156. Syria (3.069)
157. Burundi (2.905) [74]

The United States ranks number thirteen, but is separated from the happiest country, Denmark, by only a point. It is interesting to note that the bottom ten countries, including Madagascar, are in Africa, except for Syria and Afghanistan, which are both war-torn countries. Human disasters, such as the civil war occurring in Syria, call not only for humanitarian aid in terms of food and shelter, but also attention to mental health needs is required. Instead of bullets, how about Prozac?

Depression is an insidious disease, one that many may not have even considered prior to the mass attention that Prozac brought to the illness. Some call it sadness or melancholia, and depression can generally be said to range from mild to severe. But even mild depression experienced day after day is taxing and worthy of treatment. Depression now has a face that the average person can recognize, thanks to increased awareness among clinicians and the general population. Depression is also a very expensive illness, exacerbating other medical conditions and resulting in lost jobs and productivity. Depression ruins lives, and the better we understand the illness and its treatments, the happier we will be.

A Short History of Depression

The term "depression" did not appear until the mid-1800s, during a period of time when illness was a general condition most often involving a nonspecific treatment such as bloodletting or enemas. Later in the century, with the advent of bacteriology, the medical field established that indeed specific diseases had specific causes, such as the bacteria that causes cholera. This opened a door for depression to become a specific disease with a particular cause. However, following in the twentieth century, the reign of Sigmund Freud and his placement of mental illness as an internal struggle to right oneself through psychoanalysis normalized depression and other mental illnesses as "not biological." Within an increasingly cause-and-effect paradigm, there arose a mood and movement of antipsychiatry, especially during the anti-establishment 1960s, that is still active today through organizations such as the Church of Scientology. There was even a movement from within psychiatry, led by Thomas Szasz, to distance mental illness from any supposed biological causes.

> For Szasz and other 'antipsychiatrists,' mental illness should not be categorized as a disease, to be treated by therapists and psychiatrists. Szasz tried to change the definition of what was perceived as mental illness, away from biology and disruptions of the mind. The definition he wanted to prevail was outside of the field of medicine into a human condition that strikes us all as we figure out how to behave in our societies. [32]

The discovery of the SSRIs, such as Prozac, returned us to a biological view of depression, a real disease that can be treated.

Asylums and Enlightenment

But how have we arrived at psychiatry as the science of diagnosing and treating mental illnesses such as depression? Edward Shorter's *A History of Psychiatry* is a great place to start, and that text is relied on heavily in this chapter [18]. Also, the classic *Madness and Civilization* by Michel Foucault is relied upon. Whereas Shorter focuses more on the progress of treating mental illness, Foucault paints the darker side of depression using mesmerizing language, providing balance between the two works. To begin, Shorter tells us, "Before the end of the eighteenth century, there was no such thing as psychiatry" [18] and that before the nineteenth century, "looking after the insane was a family affair" [18]. Of course, before depression and other mental illnesses were isolated as diseases unto themselves, the general terms insanity and madness prevailed, but the term melancholia was also common. According to Foucault, "For a long time—until the beginning of the seventeenth century—the discussion of melancholia remained fixed within the tradition of the four humors and their essential qualities…" [58]. This remnant of the ancient Greek physician Galen spoke to the lack of progress over the centuries in recognizing the causes of mental illness.

To house and treat the insane were asylums, commonplace in the eighteenth century. According to Shorter, "All of these institutions had solely custodial functions. Traditional society had no notion of delivering therapy to patients" [18]. There were exceptions in the American colonies for "distracted persons," such as the building of private houses, "such as the five-by-seven-foot house the town of Braintree, Massachusetts, helped Samuel Speere build in 1688 to confine his insane sister, Goodwife Wittie" [18]. The first psychiatric facility was founded in Boston in 1729 with a special ward to house the insane from lesser cases.

During the eighteenth-century Enlightenment, confinement in itself became a path to curing madness. "[A] new therapeutic optimism engulfed the whole world of medicine in the second half of the eighteenth century, an optimism that psychiatry shared" [18]. But not all asylums were of a therapeutic bent. According to Foucault, "Confinement, that massive phenomenon, the signs of which are found all across eighteenth-century Europe, is a 'police matter'..." [58]. Foucault continues, noting that "at the end of the eighteenth century, all forms of madness without delirium, but characterized by inertia, by despair, by a sort of dull stupor, would be readily classifiable as melancholia" [58].

Many of the developments taken up in the United States, in what was to become the field of psychiatry, occurred overseas in France and England. It was the Parisian psychiatrist Philippe Pinel who "concluded that the asylum was a place where psychological therapy could be carried out" [18]. Pinel was famous for providing a structured day for his patients and believed that activities such as cutting wood, exercising, and painting restored the mind [18]. This bled over into British asylums and by 1837, "three-quarters of the 612 patients at Hanwell [a London asylum] were doing some kind of useful daily work" [18]. The focus was on healing the mind, foreshadowing the advent of psychotherapy. British physician John Haslam, noted for his early description of schizophrenia, said that "To achieve patients' confidence...one needed merely 'a mildness of manner and expression, an attention to their narrative, and seeming acquiescence in its truth'" [18].

These sentiments soon reached the U.S., and in 1812, Philadelphia physician Benjamin Rush, noted as the "father of American psychiatry," stated, "The cause of madness is seated primarily in the blood-vessels of the brain..." [18]. Thus, we began to understand mental illness not only as a condition of the mind but as a physical disorder located in the brain. During this time, most mental illness was either labeled as mania or melancholia, with heredity being the most common factor leading to mental illness [18].

By the 1850s, a tension arose within psychiatry between the Enlightenment, which stressed reason, and the Romantic movement, which stressed "feeling and sentiment" [18]. In *Madness and Civilization,* Foucault argues that "the notion of mental illness was a social and cultural invention of the eighteenth century" [18], albeit not a smooth innovation and one that slowly developed with research and experience on both sides of the Atlantic. Foucault says that during the nineteenth century, "Madness had become a thing to look at: no longer a monster inside oneself, but an animal with strange mechanisms, a bestiality from which man had long since been suppressed" [58]. He notes the benefits sought from cold showers and the value of travel: "The variety of the landscape dissipates the melancholic's obstinacy…" [58].

One still had to battle the idea of laziness or idleness as a cause of mental illness and had to begin considering the links with poverty as well [58]. Speaking of some French asylums, Foucault notes, "Madness was less than ever linked to medicine; nor could it be linked to the domain of correction. Unchained animality could be mastered only by discipline and brutalizing" [58]. Although there were bright spots of enlightenment, the notion of the madman languishing in a cell, rocking himself into oblivion, remained prevalent. Foucault saw progress, but odd remedies to madness remained. He relates that the Swiss physician Samuel Tissot, in the eighteenth century, had recommended eating soap to "calm many nervous ailments" [58]. The application of vinegar was also a popular treatment for madness. These basic ideas did not disappear during the nineteenth century. Shorter tells of the French physician Pierre Pomme, who believed that chicken soup and cold baths worked for symptoms such as "fatigue, pain, and a sense of dullness," which could describe depression [18].

Foucault notes the shift from barbarism, whereby force and confinement were the tools to overcome the "furies" of the mad, to more moral methods, bringing "madness and its cure into the domain of guilt" [58], a perfect platform for later psychoanalysis. Foucault quotes mid-eighteenth-century physician Francoise Leuret:

> 'Do not employ consolations, they are useless; have no recourse to reasoning, it does not persuade; do not be sad with melancholics, your sadness sustains theirs; do not assume an air of gaiety with them, they are only hurt by it. What is required is great sang froid, and when necessary, severity. Let your reason be the rule of conduct. A single string still vibrates in them, that of pain; have courage enough to pluck it.' [58]

Compassion seems very distant here, and lingering attitudes of dealing with the mentally ill brusquely have not completely disappeared.

Psychiatry and psychology as disciplines did not yet exist. Still, progress was being made toward viewing madness as a disease with specific symptoms that could be broken down into more specific categories. Foucault says of nineteenth-century practice:

> ...what had belonged to disease pertained to the organic, and what had belonged to unreason, to the transcendence of its discourse, was relegated to the psychological. And it is precisely here that psychology was born—not as the truth of madness, but as a sign that madness was now detached from its truth which was unreason and that it was

henceforth nothing but a phenomenon adrift, insignificant upon the undefined surface of nature. [58]

This phenomenon gained currency among the public as a disease that could be spread from asylums to the cities, heightening fear of the mad. Foucault notes that many asylums in Europe had been adapted from emptied leprosariums and "it was as if, across the centuries, the new tenants had received the contagion" [58].

The asylum was not unique to France or England, but was less common in the United States. Shorter says, "In 1800, only a handful of individuals were confined in asylums" [18]. In 1885, the first significant American facility for treating noninstitutionalized psychiatric patients was founded in Pennsylvania [18]. But, after the 1880s, the dismal picture of the asylum as a prison for the insane gained ground, despite efforts at understanding mental illness as a disease. Shorter notes, "After the 1880s, most American public asylums would abandon any effort at therapy… in what historian David Rothman has described as 'the decline from rehabilitation to custodianship'" [18]. By 1904, says Shorter, "there were 150,000 patients in U.S. mental hospitals" and that "by World War I, asylums had become vast warehouses for the chronically insane and demented" [18]. Why the increase in asylum patients if society was developing a more scientific outlook on mental illness? Shorter attributes this to two factors: "a 'redistribution effect' of patients being switched from family care to asylum care and a genuine increase in the rate of psychiatric illness" [18]. The more intense study of mental illness, of course, led to more people being diagnosed.

Specifically, Shorter notes that neurosyphilis contributed greatly to the rise in asylum patient numbers [18]. Shorter couples this with the rise in alcohol consumption (in the U.S.)

and refers to the nineteenth century as "the golden age of inebriation," during which consumption of alcohol went from 1.8 gallons per person per year in 1845 to 2.6 gallons in 1910 [18]. A third disease, schizophrenia, which was heavily studied in the nineteenth century, also contributed to asylum patient numbers. According to Shorter, "By 1900, psychiatry had reached a dead end" in the asylums [18], opening up opportunities to seek better forms of diagnosis and treatment.

Important to this shift, the 1880s had begun a "craze...for studying psychiatry with the microscope" in German, Austrian, and Swiss universities [18]. Unfortunately, according to Shorter, this first effort at biological psychiatry "died because it detached itself too completely from patients and their world" [18]. The research was too narrow and too finely focused on the causes versus the needs of mental health patients. What was required was a more holistic approach. But this move toward biological psychiatry would bear fruit later.

A bright spot in this close look for biological causation was the careful research of German psychiatrist Emil Kraepelin. Says Shorter, "It is Kraepelin, not Freud, who is the central figure in the history of psychiatry" [18]. Kraepelin's genius lay in collecting data on large numbers of patients and organizing them into courses of illness, which had their specific paths and outcomes [18]. By 1899, "Kraepelin's ideas reached their definitive form, resulting in a classification of illness that provided the basis of the later Diagnostic and Statistical Manual of Mental Disorders [DSM] of the American Psychiatric Association..." [18], which published its first volume in 1952.

One effect of this careful research was the development of departments of psychiatry at universities, which were "dedicated to teaching and research rather than to custodialism" [18]. Whereas Morel in the 1850s had said, "'I believe that the brain is the organ of the soul'" [18], research was placing this organ of the soul as the origin of mental illness and seeking humane ways to treat it. Although not yet entirely dissipated, tempered was the idea of punishment and confinement as the destinies of the mad.

Referencing the new attitude toward mental illness in the early twentieth century, Foucault says, "This is the moment when madness actually takes possession of confinement, while confinement itself is divested of its other forms of utility" [58]. According to Foucault, who declared asylums dead in France after the French Revolution, asylums assumed the role of "simulated family" [58], as evidenced by the compassionate work of Pinel. The asylum, though, was important in that it created a medical space for mental illness and provided physicians with the opportunity to take control of psychiatry.

Foucault calls the decline of the asylum a "moral tactic…overlaid by the myths of positivism," which fortunately were reason and logic. Foucault is cautious, though, of this seeming charity, noting that "this practice becomes more and more obscure, the psychiatrist's power more and more miraculous, and the doctor-patient couple sinks deeper into a strange world" [58], an idea that the antipsychiatry movement of the later twentieth century would embrace.

The Twentieth Century

From the advances of the nineteenth century, Shorter notes that three countries had made a significant contribution toward psychiatry: "Germany offered the first biological psychiatry, France the therapeutic asylum. The United States contributed psychoanalysis in its fullest bloom, and, latterly, much of the second biological psychiatry" [18]. In the U.S., following the escape of Sigmund Freud from Austria to the United States in 1938, the ground was fertile and receptive to his ideas of mental illness as complex sexual disorders that required a tight bonding of physician and patient. Foucault remarks, "And it is to this degree that all nineteenth-century psychiatry really converges on Freud, the first man to accept in all its seriousness the reality of the physician-patient couple" [58]. It is Freud who demystifies the asylums and places the psychiatrist at the head of the table as the key to solving mental disorders during office visits versus asylum cells.

But all was not rosy with the new century. Shorter notes that mental illness suffered from being associated with theories of degeneration, which led to forced sterilizations [18]. The rest cure, popularized during the late nineteenth century, remained popular, and asylums still existed, holding onto the past and housing the worst of the worst. Presaging Freud, Shorter furthers Foucault's recognition of the development of the doctor-patient relationship moving from the asylums to modern clinical practices, identifying "nervous illness" as the "platform for private, office-based psychiatry in the treatment of the neuroses" [18]. Private practices had no shortage of patients and were quite profitable. Shorter calls "nerves" a "fig leaf," providing the chance for psychiatrists to gracefully exit the asylums in favor of "lucrative private practice with middle-class patients" [18], which led to the ascent of doctors who called themselves neurologists. These neurologists with their private practices would soon find themselves in competition with the psychoanalysts.

Struggling, though, to establish itself as a legitimate clinical pursuit, by World War I,

> in every country in Western society psychiatry had become marginal to the mainstream of medicine…Intellectually, it was being gobbled up by medical specialties [including university departments] whose very premise was organicity. [18]

Depression Since Prozac—Finding the True Self

In other words, psychiatry was still chained to insanity, and it took someone like Freud to break that chain, even though his tenet of neurosis hinged on "fantasies of incest in childhood that opened the wellsprings of neurosis..." [18]. This was a break from the organic offerings of biological psychiatry. Says Shorter, "Freud's psychoanalysis appears as a pause in the evolution of biological approaches to brain and mind rather than as the culminating event in the history of psychiatry" [18]. But, Freud was compelling and developed a following among the middle and upper classes who could afford office visits to be analyzed, and the practice spread like a "grassfire" [18]. Furthermore, "Freud's psychoanalysis offered psychiatrists a way out of the asylum" and into mainstream society where they remain today [18].

After the 1930s, with the arrival of Freud and his followers in the U.S., the world's focus on psychiatry shifted from Europe to the U.S. [18]. The stage was set for psychoanalysis to reign, at least until the release of medications in the 1950s, such as Thorazine, Miltown, and later Prozac. With these new medications that worked wonders, psychiatry reclaimed the idea of mental illness as biological, versus being a matter of a sexually distorted mind. But, until then, "psychoanalysis flourished beyond the wildest dreams of its Viennese founders" [18].

Shorter notes a dilemma that arose in psychiatry. It became apparent that mental health patients could just be warehoused or that they could benefit from psychoanalysis, but psychoanalysis was limited to more wealthy patients and did not seek to treat "real psychiatric illness" [18]. Amid this dilemma, still there were experiments with the mentally ill, researchers trying to figure out ways to treat them. One such treatment was the fever cure, whereby patients were injected with blood tainted with malaria. Other treatments included lobotomies and immersing patients in ice water, which seemed not far from the walls of the asylum.

Thus, "Most of the twentieth century has seen restless experimentation within psychiatry to find a cure for the chronic psychoses, mainly schizophrenia and manic-depressive illness" [18].

As noted, what would prove key to biological psychiatry taking over psychoanalysis was the development of medications that actually worked against mental illness. Medications were not a new idea, but the research and rigorous trials needed to verify a drug's efficacy were unavailable. However, there were events in the past that foreshadowed later drug successes. Chloral hydrate was first described in 1832 in Germany and found to be useful as a hypnotic. Potassium bromine, first available in the 1850s, was "the first drug therapy in psychiatry that actually promised relief of psychotic illness" [18]. However, the "bromine sleep" could be toxic [18]. In 1903, barbiturates began to be used as sedatives, avoiding the toxicity of bromine. One of the first barbiturates, marketed by Bayer as Veronal, was followed by dozens more [18].

In the 1930s, two new therapies emerged: insulin coma and electroconvulsive therapy (ECT). Convulsions were induced by electric shock but also by drugs such as camphor, Cardiazol, and insulin, which patients feared because of side effects and the unpleasant experience. Although the treatments were severe, they replaced a "nihilistic hopelessness" associated with treating serious mental illness [18]. By 1959, ECT had become the treatment of choice for severe depression and generated much enthusiasm among psychiatrists [18].

In 1930, the Mental Health Treatment Act was passed in England, leading the way to open asylum doors there. This in turn fueled the community psychiatry movement in the U.S., which "ended in tragedy, the massive disgorgement of disabled asylum patients to the rough care of the streets" [18]. Thus, asylums ended as the norm, but society was not fully prepared to handle the patients formerly housed there. Looking ahead to 1946, an influential book with photographs of asylums, *The Shame of the States*, imparted the message that modern asylums were "not exactly a triumph of civilization" but rather "the greatest social debacles of our time" [18].

Psychoanalysis was all the rage in the mid-twentieth century, but the realization that mental illness was biological dented its persuasive mien. One concrete example lies within genetic studies, which evidence mental illness as a disease of the brain. Twin studies perhaps led the way in highlighting the genetic predisposition to mental illness. For example, Aaron Rosanoff in the 1930s studied 1,014 pairs of twins. Of those with schizophrenia, both twins developed the disorder in 68.3 percent of cases [18]. This sort of research debunked the fuzziness of psychoanalysis and pointed to biology. Although brain chemistry research was not new, it was pursued with increasing rigor. It was Otto Loewi who isolated the first neurotransmitter, acetylcholine, research that would lead to the discovery of the selective serotonin reuptake inhibitors (SSRIs) such as Prozac. Loewi received the Nobel Prize in 1936 for his discovery.

Other drug discoveries made their mark on the brain's chemistry as the seat of mental illness. French surgeon Henri Laborit, while experimenting with anesthetics, discovered a drug that created a revolution in psychiatry: chlorpromazine. The medication was approved by the Food and Drug Administration in 1954. An antipsychotic, marketed as Thorazine, chlorpromazine proved very effective at treating symptoms of schizophrenia. Says Shorter, "Chlorpromazine spread through the French system. 'By May 1953,' writes one historian, 'the atmosphere in the disturbed wards of mental hospitals in Paris was transformed: straitjackets...and noise were things of the past!'" [18]. According to Charles Barber, "when Thorazine was introduced at Manhattan State Psychiatric Hospital "the place transformed in a day or two from bedlam to relative calm" [22]. The discovery of chlorpromazine launched the field of modern psychopharmacology, which today holds the promise of treating most mental disorders along with psychotherapy. Shorter notes "Chlorpromazine initiated a revolution in psychiatry comparable to the introduction of penicillin in general medicine" [18].

Following in the footsteps of chlorpromazine came a wide variety of antipsychotic, antimanic, and antidepressant drugs. The effect changed "psychiatry from a branch of social work to a field that called for the most precise knowledge of pharmacology, the effect of drugs on the body" [18], which included the discovery of the tranquilizer Miltown in 1955. "Like Prozac in the 1990s, Miltown became a pop culture phenomenon" [44]. Another groundbreaking drug, lithium, was discovered by John Cade to treat mania, the first studies being conducted in 1960.

The First Antidepressants

By 1960, three antidepressants were available: isoniazid (also a treatment for tuberculosis), imipramine (a TCA or tricyclic antidepressant), and iproniazid (a monoamine oxidase inhibitor or MAOI). Although the medications seemed effective, it was unclear why they worked. But by the late 1960s, a "seemingly logical story had developed," indicating that neurotransmitters processed the brain's electrical impulses. [18] In 1952, Betty Twarog identified serotonin as a neurotransmitter [18]. Later, in the 1970s, researchers would ask if low serotonin was a symptom or cause of depression, leading to the discovery and use of the SSRIs such as Prozac.

The first modern antidepressant, isoniazid, appeared in the early 1950s. First used to treat tuberculosis and then investigated by psychiatrist Nathan Kline, the drug seemed a wonder, but it had a nasty side effect of creating jaundice, and the manufacturer pulled back. But, according to von Praag, "the psychotropic agents were revolutionizing psychiatry" [59].

According to Hillhouse and Porter, regarding isoniazid, "serendipity played an important role in the discovery of the first pharmacological treatment for depression" [77]. Intrigued with the drug, chemists then experimented and discovered iproniazid, which had side effects that included euphoria, psychostimulation, increased appetite, and improved sleep [77]. This led to further research that led to the discovery of imipramine (Tofranil) by Roland Kuhn, the first drug specifically developed to fight depression. Kuhn found that imipramine "produced marked improvements in patients suffering from severe depression" [77], that the response was "'absolutely incredible, so exciting'" [18]. Thus, the drug industry had a new class of highly profitable medications on its hands and sought to make more.

Antipsychiatry

In the 1960s, one negative result of the new medications involved the emptying of psychiatric hospitals as patients became manageable with medication. As with the emptying of asylums earlier in the twentieth century, the discovery of these new medications produced a "massive discharge of psychiatric patients to the 'community,' a process known as deinstitutionalization..." [18]. According to Shorter, in the U.S., the number of those institutionalized went from 559,000 in 1955 to 107,000 by 1988, a reduction of 80 percent, which Shorter describes as "the greatest debacle of twentieth-century psychiatry" [18]. Shorter notes that the National Institute of Mental Health, created by the Mental Health Act in 1946, was partly responsible for the shift that led to the creation of community health centers, engineered by John F. Kennedy's 1963 Community Mental Health Act. The centers were unable to manage the newly released, and many patients became homeless and worse. This migration of patients out of the system played well into the hands of the antipsychiatry movement and their "rage" against psychiatry [18]. According to Shorter, antipsychiatrists and the community psychiatry movement preached "a romanticized vision of welcoming friends and neighbors clasping the mentally ill to their bosoms" [18], which did not happen.

A shift from the short-lived community psychiatry, which had evolved from asylum psychiatry, to corporate psychiatry characterized the 1960s [22]. This new corporate psychiatry, with its successful new medications, did not earn trust from many, though, especially among psychoanalysts whose livelihood was being threatened, and the antipsychiatry movement gained momentum. "The availability of specific medications for psychosis and depression made diagnosis a practical matter" [18], defusing the psychoanalyst's modus operandi of mental illness as seated in complexes versus being diseases with concrete treatments. The publication of *The Myth of Mental Illness* in 1961 by psychoanalyst Thomas Szasz characterized psychiatry as "scientifically worthless and socially harmful" [18]. In fiction, an influential book proved to be Ken Kesey's *One Flew Over the Cuckoo's Nest*, published in 1962. According to Shorter, the book's message was this: "Psychiatric patients are not ill, they're merely deviant" [18]. Another facet of antipsychiatry was the rise of Scientology under the leadership of L. Ron Hubbard, who declared psychiatrists as evil and cited psychiatry as abusive. Thus, the tension between the evolving psychiatry establishment and antipsychiatry was very real. Shorter describes it this way:

> By the end of the 1960s, the antipsychiatric interpretation of 'so-called psychiatric illness' had gained the catbird seat among intellectuals both in the United States and in Europe. In these circles, a consensus had formed that the discipline of psychiatry was an illegitimate form of social control and that psychiatrists' power to lock people up

must be abolished... [18]

Narrow in scope and weak in clinical advice, the second edition of the *DSM*, which was to become the "Bible" of psychiatry with the third edition, appeared in 1968, reflecting what psychiatry lacked at the time: research-based diagnoses paired with empirically proven treatments. Shorter says, "In the 1960s, the discipline began to wake up to the importance of getting the diagnosis right" [18]. This new generation of psychiatrists "determined that psychiatry should proceed as the rest of medicine did, establishing a differential diagnosis based on presenting symptoms, then conducting a proper investigation to come up with a clinical diagnosis..." [18]. Armed with medications and diagnostic criteria, psychiatry moved forward, pushing past the resistance, now holding hands with the pharmaceutical industry. According to David Healey, a pivotal development was the 1962 Food and Drug Act amendments, enacted in response to the thalidomide debacle, "which channeled drug development toward clear diseases" [51]. This was a healthy response and girded the position of psychiatry against the antipsychiatry movement, which ultimately did not have the large-scale social setting needed to receive it [49].

The Revival of Biological Psychiatry

In the 1970s, the antipsychiatry movement waned as "biological psychiatry came roaring back on stage, displacing psychoanalysis as the dominant paradigm and returning psychiatry to the fold of the other medical specialties" [18] versus being a pseudoscience. With the grip of psychoanalysis further weakened, mental illness became medicalized and treatable through medical means" [18]. Shorter notes, "By the 1990s, a majority of psychiatrists considered psychoanalysis scientifically bankrupt" [18]. Van Praag adds:

> [T]he biological revolution in psychiatry was accompanied by a renewed interest in the diagnosis, differential diagnosis, and assessment of abnormal behavior. Biological psychiatry is the single most important factor in the revival of psychopathological research... [59]

This new precision of psychiatry boded well for the development of the new antidepressants, the SSRIs, such as Prozac. Since the 1960s, evidence had been mounting that serotonin played a significant role in depression. Big pharma company Eli Lilly took the lead in developing a medication to increase brain serotonin, and in 1974, the first report on a new drug, fluoxetine (Prozac), was published. Released in 1987, Prozac was a drug that psychiatrists and general practitioners could safely prescribe for an increasingly widespread illness. Perhaps as a result of intense marketing or an intense need, Shorter notes that "The boundaries of what constitutes depression [were] expanded relentlessly outward," which soon led to depression becoming "the single commonest disorder seen in psychiatric practice" [18]. In a practical vein, with the rise of antidepressants, the eagerness to treat depression rose. As physicians like to diagnose conditions they can treat, the number of depressed people and those thus treated increased. Considering self-interest, Shorter notes that psychiatrists "pushed the boundary of pathology steadily to the right, away from the unwell and to the commonplace," which represented billable psychiatric illnesses [18], and thus an affirmation of corporate psychiatry. With this rise in patient numbers also came an increase in the number of private psychiatric hospitals in the United States, from 150 in 1970 to 444 in 1988 [18].

In concert with the new medications were the clinical trials required by the Food and Drug Administration to approve them. The rigorous clinical trial procedure, precipitated by the global thalidomide disaster in the early 1960s, was put into action through the 1962 Drug Amendments, which bolstered legislation going back to 1938. Only 10 percent of medications undergoing clinical trials receive FDA approval. Clinical trials added a new twist in the legal sphere. Patients and their lawyers expected to receive medications that worked, based on empirical evidence.

This claim to efficacious treatment is shown best by the case of "Osheroff versus Chestnut Lodge," which began with the admittance of Raphael Osheroff to Chestnut Lodge, originally established as a sanitarium to treat alcoholics and those with nervous disorders [78]. Osheroff was diagnosed with a variety of symptoms, including depression and suicidal thoughts. The Lodge treated him with psychotherapy and withheld medications. Osheroff's condition worsened, and he lost his medical license and custody of his two children in the process. Osheroff sued, claiming that effective medicines had been available, but that they had been denied him, and he settled the lawsuit in 1987 for an undisclosed amount. Says Kramer, "Osheroff was enormously influential. Hospital administrators understood that their institutions would be at legal risk if their staff withheld medications whose worth had been demonstrated in clinical trials" [23].

Another tangle in the knot of psychiatry was the rise in the number of practicing psychologists. By the 1990s, clinical psychologists and social workers outnumbered psychiatrists, basically rendering psychiatry a "nonmedical activity" [18]. This, of course, bred competition. Shorter observes that psychiatrists pathologize human behavior to make medical treatments viable. He states that psychiatrists "have been willing to draw the pathology line ever lower in their efforts to tear as much counseling as possible away from competing psychologists and social workers" [18]. In 1995, psychologists lobbied Congress for the prescribing privilege, and the American Psychiatric Association successfully lobbied Congress with vigor to withhold this privilege from psychologists; this remains in effect today [18]. Psychiatrists, along with nurse practitioners and physician assistants under their direct supervision, hold the keys to prescribing medications.

Throughout the rest of the 1990s, depression as a diagnosis and topic of research soared. Doing a Medline search for major depression, Dan Blazer found an astonishing rise in the number of hits from 1975, when there were no hits, to 1,224 hits in 2000 [57]. That number now stands at 868, indicating that some forward momentum may have been lost, but research remains active. Despite the quandaries of psychiatry as a discipline and what Barber calls "corporate psychiatry," the range of treatment options for the depressed, especially regarding medications such as the SSRIs, is wide. According to Kramer,

> The personality of the new medications—ease in prescribing, relative safety in overdose, social acceptability, and favorable impact on social functioning—[has] allowed for the spread of mental health care at a level with little precedent. [23]

That's great news for those being treated, but more efforts are needed to reach those still in need of treatment.

From the bowels of asylum care and an increasing awareness of mental illness as a biological entity, depression slowly emerged as a diagnosis unto itself. With the discovery of the neurotransmitters, effective treatments in the form of antidepressants emerged in the 1950s. Gone were the asylums. Clinicians now saw patients in their offices and treated them with medications proven effective in clinical trials. From this, Prozac emerged and changed the course of depression from a remnant of madness into a common psychiatric disorder as defined by the *DSM*.

Sweet Serotonin

What is serotonin, and why do we need it? Basically, neurons in the brain communicate with one another using neurotransmitters such as serotonin. A signal is released, carried by the serotonin to the next neuron, and then the serotonin is absorbed. SSRIs block the reuptake of serotonin, increasing its availability for brain function.

A new class of medications, known as selective serotonin reuptake inhibitors (SSRIs), officially appeared with the release of Prozac in 1987, although the first SSRI, zimelidine, was developed in 1972. The discovery of serotonin and its role in depression has effectively re-legitimized psychiatrists as the gatekeepers of mental illness, specifically depression, nearly taking it from the hands of psychoanalysts and psychologists who cannot prescribe medications unless trained as medical doctors. Not only could psychiatrists firmly claim depression, but they had a treatment, the SSRIs, that the pharmaceutical industry so willingly provided. According to David Wong et al., "the success of fluoxetine [Prozac] has heightened awareness of depression, underscored the crucial need for treatment and reduced the stigma associated with the disorder" [66].

Edward Shorter, in his definitive *A History of Psychiatry*, traces the discovery of the first neurotransmitter, acetylcholine, back to Otto Loewi in the early 1920s [18]. In the 1930s, acetylcholine was given to schizophrenic patients, but without result. Broadly, the three major neurotransmitters—serotonin, norepinephrine, and dopamine—are known as monoamines. According to Tod Hillhouse and Joseph Porter, "The monoamine hypothesis proposes that patients with depression have depleted concentrations of serotonin, norepinephrine, and dopamine" [77]. Serotonin levels are determined by measuring 5-HIAA levels, the technical term for the serotonin metabolite that results once serotonin is used. According to M.T. Walsh and T.G. Dinan,

> It has been recognized since the early 1970s that reduced levels of 5-HIAA in CSF [cerebrospinal fluid] often occurs in depression...It was recognized subsequently that in depressed patients with low 5-HIAA there were significantly more suicide attempters than in patients with normal 5-HIAA... [79]

By the late 1980s, the role of serotonin (5-HT) in depression and suicide began to receive revived attention. J.J. Mann et al. examined studies of 5-HT and 5-HIAA among suicide victims going back to 1969. They discovered a significant reduction of serotonin and its metabolite in tissue from brain stems, frontal cortices, and other areas of the brain. It is the role of antidepressants to block 5-HT binding sites, making more serotonin available for synaptic functions, influencing depression and suicidal ideation/acts. Kramer also notes, "A variety of postmortem studies have compared the brains of otherwise physically healthy people who died from suicide with those who died as accident victims. What distinguishes the suicides is low levels of brain serotonin" [23].

Brain serotonin levels are not routinely measured because collecting cerebrospinal fluid requires an invasive procedure. Serotonin can be measured in the blood, with platelets accounting for 90 percent of circulating serotonin, but this does not reflect brain serotonin levels. Serotonin allows communication between neurons not only in the brain but throughout the body, and many, if not most, of the serotonin receptors are found in the intestines [80]. This may explain some of the gastrointestinal side effects of the SSRIs, such as nausea or queasiness.

The research behind the development of the monoamine hypothesis, which correlates low levels of serotonin with depression, is summarized well by Hillhouse and Porter [77]. According to them: "Two primary lines of evidence led to the development of the monoamine hypothesis: 1) the effects of reserpine on serotonin and catecholamines; and 2) the pharmacological mechanisms of action of antidepressant drugs" [77]. When reserpine was used as an antihypertensive, it was noted that the reserpine caused depression in some patients [77]. Once removed from reserpine, the depressive symptoms abated. It was discovered that reserpine depleted brain monoamines such as serotonin, giving evidence for the depleted neurotransmitters being a cause of depression [77]. They do note, however, that other research indicates that depletion of serotonin in healthy subjects does not produce depressive symptoms [77]. Thus, one must be prone to depression as a result of depleted neurotransmitters, hinting at genetic factors potentially at play. Or, as Hillhouse and Porter note, depleted monoamines "must be present in the context of stressors" [77] to precipitate depression.

Citing the work of other researchers, Hillhouse and Porter note that there are patients who do not respond to any antidepressant agents, suggesting that low brain serotonin levels may be part of a larger neurobiological system rather than a direct cause of depression [77]. This means that serotonin and other neurotransmitters are important indicators of depression, but that not all of the weight of the disease can be attributed to them. This has led to research aimed at revising the monoamine hypothesis and seeking other brain receptor targets that are not monoamines. One promising research focus has focused on the glutamatergic system [77].

Glutamate is a neurotransmitter, similar to serotonin, but

is not a monoamine. Glutamate is much more prevalent in the brain than serotonin and is "the major excitatory neurotransmitter and makes functional contributions to more than half of all synapses in the brain" [77]. According to Mark J. Niciu et al., "the glutamate system contributes to the pathophysiology of major mood disorders, including major depressive disorder (MDD)" [81]. Thus, as the primary excitatory neurotransmitter in our central nervous system, [81] glutamate shows great promise as a mechanism to possibly alleviate depression. One application of treating the glutamatergic system involves ketamine, an anesthetic. In one study, within four hours, ketamine produced rapid antidepressant effects that lasted up to 72 hours as compared to placebo [77].

Prior to the SSRIs, we primarily had two classes of medications to treat depression, the tricyclic antidepressants (TCAs) and monoamine oxidase inhibitors (MAOIs). These medications also work to boost neurotransmitters but come with some serious side effects if not used with caution. TCAs may cause blurred vision, dizziness, constipation, and dry mouth. MAOIs mix badly with certain foods that contain tyramine, such as processed meats and cheeses. According to Wong et al., "[O]verall, the ease of use, safety and relatively benign side effects of fluoxetine [Prozac] have led to better patient acceptance, compliance and outcomes." SSRIs such as Prozac can be taken once a day, and the dosage range is easy to arrive at based on the level of depression, which doctors appreciate. According to Wong et al., "Psychiatrists now have a safe, effective and well-tolerated armamentarium in fluoxetine [Prozac] and other SSRIs for the treatment of this severe mental illness" [66].

Increasing serotonin treats the symptoms of depression but also has beneficial side effects. According to Michael J. Norden, "Serotonin and its chief metabolite...melatonin, protect organisms from 'oxidative stress,' the biological equivalent of rusting" [28]. Norden also reports that "studies show that drugs that increase serotonin activity lessen aggression, while those that reduce serotonin activity heighten aggression" [28]. But this does not mean that serotonin will make you a doormat. In a study involving vervet monkeys, "[I]n every instance the high-serotonin male was the dominant male in the troop" [23]. One aspect of reducing depression is increasing one's self-confidence and being in control of one's life. Kramer adds,

> However low self-worth is acquired, a medication that raises serotonin levels might move a person biochemically from the feelings of subordinate status toward the feelings and even the behaviors of dominant status. [23]

A good thing, although critics such as Charles Barber, Joseph Glenmullen, and Eric Wilson would decry this as an unnatural or unfair advantage [22, 25, 26].

Norden discusses an interesting aspect of serotonin regarding sunlight. He says that, being previously creatures who spent much time outside, our brains evolved in the presence of daily sunlight and the rhythms of seasons. [28]. Norden is an advocate of light therapy, the light boxes that many with depression use, and says that "light stimulates the brain as surely as Prozac..." [28]. A metabolite of serotonin is melatonin, which many take as a sleep aid. According to Norden, "melatonin dysfunction plays a part in the type of depression known as melancholia," and "insomniacs had a forty-fold increased risk of developing major depression" [28]. Not only can sleep deprivation result from a lack of serotonin, but also "sleep deprivation can produce a 20 percent decrease in brain serotonin" [28]. Thus, one can take SSRIs such as Prozac and receive similar benefits that sunlight brings, which is a necessary adjunct therapy for depressives. Another treatment for depression, which raises serotonin levels, is exercise. Norden reports that 90 minutes on a treadmill doubles brain serotonin levels [28]. Those who exercise know well "the melting away of tension and aggression that exercise provides" [28].

So, raising one's serotonin levels is conducive to decreasing depression, as proven by clinical and trial data. It is also crucial that those with depression engage in other activities that stimulate serotonin levels, such as getting outside into the sunlight, sleeping well, and exercising.

Side Effects of Increasing Serotonin

No drug comes without side effects, including the SSRIs like Prozac. Warnings and precautions, as noted on the prescribing information for Prozac, include: allergic reaction and rash, activation of mania/hypomania, seizures, abnormal bleeding, glaucoma, hyponatremia, anxiety, insomnia, potential for cognitive and motor impairment, and most notably, the black-box warning for suicidal thoughts and behaviors for children, teenagers, and young adults [82]. It is thought that those who are depressed often lack the energy to think of suicide or carry through with a plan, and that being lifted from their funk suddenly can carry out self-harm. However, "Though the suggestion has been made that fluoxetine [Prozac] may trigger an emotional state which itself increases the risk of suicide, this suggestion has not been supported by formal evidence" [83]. The important topic of suicide in general and the impact of SSRIs on suicidal thoughts and behaviors is discussed in chapter nine.

Thus, taking Prozac and other medications like it comes with risks, but the risks listed above seem minimal. For example, in clinical trials, dry mouth occurred in 10 out of 1,728 patients being treated with Prozac for depression [82]. Other side effects that may also be considered rare are nausea, diarrhea, anorexia, nervousness, abnormal dreams, and yawning [82].

Sexual Dysfunction

Among those who take Prozac and medications like it, the occurrence of decreased libido, or sexual dysfunction, may be the most powerful reason why someone would choose not to take the drug or decide to discontinue the drug. According to Norden, "Far and away the most common side effect [of Prozac]...is sexual dysfunction" [28]. Elizabeth Wurtzel highlights this saying, "This seemed to be a routine for me, getting started on sexual encounters and not only stopping them, but actually fleeing from the room as if in shame or in danger..." [27]. Anna Moore lightheartedly calls this sexual dysfunction "one of Prozac's hidden extras" [17], but very real to many who take Prozac and other SSRIs. Moore goes as far as to say, "SSRIs could seriously impede our ability to fall and stay in love" [17]. But this sexual dysfunction is not unique to the SSRIs and occurs with other classes of antidepressants as well.

An interesting upside to this lack of desire to have sex concerns persons with disorders that are considered sexually deviant. Lauren Slater gives us this about Bill, who was addicted to sex: "'Listen,' he says, 'sex is dead. It's dead,' he says, briefly patting his crotch like it is a pet. 'It's gone'" [84]. Slater quotes Martin Kafka, who treats paraphilia, a type of sexual perversion:

> It used to be thought sexual deviants had just testosterone abnormalities, but they may really have serotonin abnormalities. It may be that the lower the serotonin, the higher the sex drive, or it may be something much more complex, that sexual deviance is linked to an as yet unidentified disregulation in the serotonin system. [84]

Thus, for those with sex drives that are unreasonable or that endanger others, the SSRIs seem to be an effective treatment.

Ultimately, receiving treatment is a choice. The side effects of Prozac are not guaranteed, but the action of increasing serotonin available to the brain comes with possible trade-offs. For those dogged by depression, the risk of suicidal thoughts, yawning, or decreased libido may very well be worth it. There is one antidepressant, Wellbutrin (buproprion), that does seem to have the lowest risk of sexual dysfunction [77].

Low levels of serotonin and other neurotransmitters have been proven to be associated with depression and suicide. Medications such as Prozac make more of that serotonin available to the brain, reducing depressive symptoms and hopefully saving lives. There is an initial danger that the medications will increase suicidal thoughts, and patients need to be aware of that. On a firm foundation with serotonin, researchers are looking to other neurotransmitters, such as glutamate, to refine theories of causation and seek even better medications. Prozac and the SSRIs do not come without side effects, the most serious perhaps being sexual dysfunction. But one must weigh the agony of depression with side effects and make a choice.

The Rise of Prozac

Beginning with Prozac (fluoxetine) in 1987, forming a new class of antidepressants, the SSRIs took the world by storm, especially in the United States. Prozac took on a life of its own, and an unprecedented flow of popular and medical literature praised it and railed against it. According to K. Sharpe, the "SSRIs were an A-list topic of debate in the culture wars, and the rhetoric, whether pro or con, was red hot" [38]. According to M. Olfson et al., "the growth in antidepressant use was greatest after fluoxetine hydrochloride [Prozac] first became available in late 1987" [85]. But the meteoric rise in its popularity had been in rehearsal perhaps since the 1850s when chloral hydrate, the first drug aimed at treating mental illness, gained a popular following. Amphetamines arrived in the late 1880s. No new major discoveries would be made until 1943 with the discovery of the mind-altering LSD, which failed to find a useful application in psychiatry. The 1950s were banner years, though, with the introduction first of the antipsychotic chlorpromazine (Thorazine), followed successively by the first three antidepressants: isoniazid, imipramine, and iproniazid.

Much research on brain chemistry has been conducted since 1900, culminating in the discovery of the first neurotransmitter, acetylcholine, by Otto Loewi in the 1920s. In 1952, Betty Twarog identified serotonin as a neurotransmitter. According to Edward Shorter, 1953 marked the rise of serotonin as a solution to depression, setting the stage for Prozac. Shorter quotes John Gaddum, a psychopharmacologist of the period, as saying "'It is possible that the 5-HT [serotonin] in our brains plays an essential part in keeping us sane'" [18]. By 1955, a new drug, Miltown (meprobamate), was sweeping the nation. It lifted "quotidian anxiety and depression," and had few side effects, another foreshadowing of Prozac [18]. After rumors and gossip of this new wonder drug circulated at the annual American Psychiatric Association meeting, the demand for Miltown "was far greater than for any drug ever marketed in the United States" [18]. The demand was so high that drug stores would run out and post signs in their windows announcing when more would be available.

By 1959, although the new antidepressants were gaining some ground, "ECT [electroconvulsive therapy] had become 'the treatment of choice'...for manic-depressive illness and major depression" [18], and ECT remains today as an effective treatment for depression that is unresponsive to medication. In 1960, a new wonder drug emerged, Librium (chlordiazepoxide). The first of the benzodiazepines to be marketed, the drug became the best-selling prescription drug in the United States [18]. Due to side effects, though, the manufacturer of Librium, Roche, sought a new benzodiazepine and developed Valium (diazepam), "which until the introduction of Prozac was the single most successful drug in pharmaceutical history" [18]. Says Shorter, "As Valium soared in popularity, awareness dawned among drug makers that here lay the markets of the future" [18]. This occurred with the rise of the first-generation antidepressants, the tricyclic antidepressants (TCAs), which are "the number one cause of emergency room visits for overdose toxicity" [28] and monoamine oxidase inhibitors (MAOIs), which interact toxically with foods containing tyramine, being famous for the cheese reaction [28].

The 1970s produced the research needed to get Prozac up and running. According to David T. Wong et al., "In the early 1970s, evidence of the role of serotonin...in depression began to emerge and the hypothesis that enhancing 5-HT neurotransmission would be a viable mechanism to mediate antidepressant response was put forward" [66]. In 1973, Wong et al. approached Eli

Depression Since Prozac—Finding the True Self

Lilly with their findings, and a project team was formed to guide the new drug through product development. Prozac's initial moniker was LY110141. According to the developers,

> We first disclosed our pharmacological studies of fluoxetine in a series of oral presentations at the 1974 annual meetings of the Federation of American Societies for Experimental Biology and the American Society of Pharmacology and Experimental Therapeutics…[W]e proposed that fluoxetine [Prozac] would be a potential antidepressant drug. [66]

Phase I of the clinical trial was successful but ran into problems in Phase II, the trial showing that Prozac "was found to be ineffective" [66]. The researchers were disappointed but pressed on, concluding that their trial patients "had previously been found to be refractory to other antidepressive treatments" [66]. Phase III, though, proved successful and "expeditiously brought the trials to a definitive and successful conclusion." Prozac proved to be effective in the treatment of major depression.

By 1999, Prozac sales accounted for 25 percent of Eli Lilly's $10 billion in revenue [17]. Interbrand, a leading global branding company, created the name Prozac. Following clinical trials, which proved Prozac's efficacy, Prozac was released for marketing in December 1987. Says Wong et al.,

> To many of us, the news brought not only excitement, but also an ultimate vindication, as we had carried the burden of the project, and had been ridiculed for many years as the ones who discovered and developed a molecule looking for a disease. [66]

This criticism of disease mongering remains.

The effects of Prozac on depression and on psychiatric practice were unprecedented. According to Shorter, "The share of psychiatric patients receiving prescriptions increased from a quarter of all office visits in 1975 to fully one-half by 1990" [18], much of this increase attributed to Prozac and medications like it. By 1990, Prozac was the number one drug prescribed by psychiatrists [18].

As Prozac gained traction in the 1980s, the number of psychiatric office visits in which an antidepressant was prescribed soared from 23.1 percent in 1985 to 48.6 percent in 1993–1994 [85]. Olfson et al. also found that "psychiatric patients were approximately 2.3...times more likely to receive an antidepressant in 1993–1994 than in 1985" and that "between 1980 and 1989, annual prescriptions of antidepressants by office-based physicians in the United States increased from 10 to 13.2 million. The fastest growth occurred among prescriptions written by psychiatrists" [85]. By 1991, Prozac was the best-selling antidepressant, with sales approaching $1 billion per year [25]. By 2002, "Prozac had been prescribed to more than 40 million patients worldwide with total sales of US $22 billion; the peak annual sales were US $2.8 billion in 1998" [66]. By 2007, Prozac was prescribed to 54 million people worldwide [17].

Office visits for depression continued to rise through the early 1990s, nearly doubling from 10.99 million in 1988 to 20.43 million in 1993 and 1994 [86]. Between 1990 and 2000, antidepressant use quadrupled [23]. Continuing to rise in popularity, Prozac and medications like it infiltrated the popular mind and scientific media. By 2013, it was famously reported that "one in six U.S. adults reported taking a psychiatric drug, such as an antidepressant or a sedative..." [87]. From that same survey, as reported by Moore, "Antidepressants were the most common type of psychiatric drug in the survey, with 12 percent of adults reporting that they filled prescriptions for these drugs" [87]. Eli Lilly's Prozac patent expired in 2001, costing them $35 million in market share in a single day [17]. Although Prozac was taking a back seat to its cousin SSRIs and generics, it remained a primary drug in the public eye. By 2013, Prozac had relinquished the top spot, and two new antidepressants succeeded Prozac: sertraline hydrochloride (Zoloft) and citalopram hydrobromide (Celexa) [87].

Much has been made of big pharma and its role in marketing antidepressants. The drug companies developing and selling antidepressants certainly have spent a lot of money getting the word out about their products. According to Elliott, "the industry has learned that the key to selling psychiatric drugs is to sell the illnesses they treat" [39]. He cites the case of Merck and amitriptyline in the early 1960s. Merck distributed 50,000 copies of "Recognizing the Depressed Patient" [39], which encouraged clinicians to find and treat depression with their drug. Another spending opportunity is the annual National Depression Screening Day, funded by pharmaceutical companies through Mental Health America (MHA). According to the Citizens Commission on Human Rights International (CCHR),

> their [MHA] 2007 Annual Report showed the slush fund continued: Lilly, Bristol-Myers Squibb, and Wyeth gave $1 million or more. Janssen and Pfizer donated between $500,000 to $999,999. AstraZeneca and Forest gave between $100,000 and $499,999, while GSK increased its donation to between $50,000 and $99,999, along with the Pharmaceutical Research and Manufacturers of America. Otsuka America Pharmaceutical, Shire US and Solvay gave ($10,000 to $24,999). [88]

Corporate funding for 2016 made up 40 percent of MHA's revenue [89]. Of course, screening for depression is not a bad idea, especially if you have an effective treatment to accompany it. It just looks like the drug companies are out to beat the bushes for potential customers. From a business standpoint, it makes sense, and if people are truly helped, then it is hard to criticize the revenue. A cost that many sometimes forget about is the development cost of a drug, money that must be recouped through sales. According to Michael Norden, to bring a new drug to market can cost roughly $150 to $250 million [28]. Thus, big pharma risks hundreds of millions of dollars and must profit to survive, like any business that invests in the future.

There is much other data to support the rise in popularity of the SSRIs, such as Prozac, and the rise in the number of people seeking psychiatric treatment for illnesses such as depression. In 2014, mental health expenditures were $186 billion [90]. It is interesting to note that, from 1986 to 2014, inpatient mental health costs decreased from 41 percent to 16 percent of total mental health expenditures, while prescription medications increased from 8 percent to 27 percent [90]. In 2014, antidepressants overall ranked third in sales, only topped by analgesics and cholesterol-lowering medications [91]. According to Laura Pratt, Debra Brody, and Qiuping Gu,

> Antidepressants were the third most common prescription drug taken by Americans of all ages in 2005–2008 and the most frequently used by persons aged 18–44 years. From 1988–1994 through 2005–2008, the rate of antidepressant use in the United States among all ages increased nearly 400 percent...Twenty-three percent of women aged 40–59 take antidepressants, more than in any other age-sex group. [92]

Continuing into 2014, for which the latest published data is available, there were 41,498,000 psychiatric office visits in 2014, and 7,820,000 (19 percent) of those visits were for depression [91]. A diagnosis of depression was recorded at 10.3 percent of all office visits, with women at 12.7 percent and men at 7 percent [91]. Overall, at all office visits, 142,674,000 mentions of antidepressants were made, making up 4.5 percent of all drug mentions at all office visits, although the most mentioned psychiatric drug was Alprazolam, an anxiolytic [91]. Some good news about psychiatric office visits is that psychiatry ranked highest in average office visit length, at 34.8 minutes [91].

There are various ways to explain this rise of Prozac and the SSRIs. Perhaps Olfson et al. explain it best:

> In the last few years, several developments have focused renewed attention on patterns of antidepressant use. First, the armamentarium of antidepressant medications has continued to expand as newer selective serotonin reuptake inhibitors (SSRIs) and antidepressants with atypical mechanisms of action have become available, beginning with fluoxetine [Prozac] in late 1987. Second, there has been a surge in public interest in antidepressants. Fluoxetine and other newer antidepressants have been the topic of lead articles in national news magazines, best-selling books, and widely watched television talk shows. Third, drug companies have begun to market antidepressants and other prescription medications on television and in the lay press. Fourth, antidepressants are clinically useful in an expanding range of psychiatric and general medical disorders. [85]

Also, as widely reported, SSRIs have fewer toxic side effects than first-generation antidepressants (TCAs and MAOIs) and are less dangerous in the hands of someone who may become suicidal [85]. SSRIs have not completely displaced the first-generation antidepressants, but the public knows them best. SSRIs have also been found helpful in treating other disorders such as anxiety and eating disorders, widening market appeal. Another key development has been the "shifting attitudes regarding depression" [93]. Thanks to Prozac and the SSRIs, depression has become a household term, and people are less afraid to identify themselves as depressed and less fearful of seeking treatment.

The evolution of Prozac from idea to product took 16 years, and the medication became wildly popular. When Foucault said "...the subject must be restored to his initial purity, and must be wrested from his pure subjectivity in order to be initiated into the world..." [58], he had no idea how a single medication would do just that. Foucault also said, "What is wanted, then, is a cure that will give the spirits or the fibers a vigor, but a calm vigor, a strength no disorder can mobilize..." [58]. Prozac is not a cure for depression, but the term "calm vigor" seems to resonate with the SSRIs, and according to Moore, "Prozac hit a society that was in the mood for it...It was the wonder drug, the easy answer, an instant up..." [17].

Today, the Prozac phenomenon has waned, but it is indelibly inscribed in American and global consciousness. According to K. Sharpe, "Like the automobile or the telephone before them, SSRIs are a one-time miracle technology that have since become a familiar—even frumpy—part of the furniture of modern life" [38]. Kimberly K. Emmons says of Prozac, "[T]he brand name has been used by memoirists and scholars alike as a metonym for depression itself..." [56]. Thus, Prozac and depression have become intertwined, much as Oscar Meyer is synonymous with hot dogs. Emmons examines the phenomenon, saying,

> The discourse of depression draws heavily on pharmaceutical interventions that seek to promise simple cures. The historically recent and relatively unprecedented popular

usage of psychotropic drugs serves as an indication of our collective entry into what Lawrence Rubin calls 'the new asylum,' a place where the walls of confinement are invisible... [56]

Emmons highlights the effect of the SSRIs on a move from hospitalizing patients, which began in the 1960s, toward outpatient treatment with medications, which is a good thing for those suffering from an easily treated illness. Prozac, in essence, makes us feel better and gives us that push we need. There is no need to be locked up. In a humorous tone, Mary Leonard says,

Of all the cultural markers of the last 10 years—the Internet, the Simpsons, gourmet coffee shops—none has made us feel better than Prozac. A wonder drug for depression and a low-risk prescription, Prozac enters its second decade as a household word and not just mother's little helper. Grandpa acting grumpy? Benji barking his head off? Little Susie feeling sad? Put them on Prozac. [94]

Those sentiments remain to this day, but the news about Prozac was not always positive, some claiming that Prozac worked no better than placebo, and some decrying its potential to unleash violent behavior, which is addressed in chapter six, "Prozac under Fire."

The Cost of Prozac

Regarding overall spending on medications in the U.S., in 2013, "per capita spending on prescription drugs was $858 compared with an average of $400 for 19 other industrialized nations" [95]. We spend twice as much per person. So, how much do antidepressants actually cost? This is easy to find by looking at online providers of medication costs, such as GoodRx.com, which lists medications by class and shows retail prices at various outlets, including Walmart, CVS, and Walgreens. Regarding Prozac (fluoxetine), the lowest price is around $4.00 at Walmart [96]. This is for a 30-day supply. The low price for Paxil is $9. One of the most expensive antidepressant is Pexeva at $405. Interestingly—and perhaps not surprisingly—Walmart most often offers the lowest price [96]. Looking at the older antidepressants, prices are much higher than the SSRIs. For a 30-day supply of MAOIs, the prices range from $39 for Nardil to $1,691 for Emsam. For TCAs, the prices range from $9 for Pamelor to $420 for Silenor. Imipramine (Tofranil), a TCA and the first drug manufactured specifically for depression, is still on the market at $10 for a 30-day supply.

Looking at *Consumer Reports,* which rates and provides cost data on a variety of products, there are no costs or rankings, and the site is unable to judge the medications' qualitative and quantitative aspects. Surprisingly, the site downplays medications as a treatment, saying, "In studies, roughly 30 to 50 percent of people with moderate to severe depression aren't helped at all with the initial antidepressant treatment" [82]. The report suggests trying cognitive behavioral therapy before trying antidepressants.

Although big pharma serves many good purposes, developing and marketing effective medications such as Prozac, there are examples of sheer greed. Perhaps the most egregious in recent history concerns the drug Daraprim, which is used to treat infections usually seen in patients with HIV/AIDS. In 2015, the medication went from $13.50 per tablet to $750 per tablet, making annual treatment cost hundreds of thousands for a single patient. The drug was originally developed by GlaxoSmithKline but was later licensed to CorePharma. At that point, a single tablet went from $1 to $13.50. Then Turing licensed the drug, and the price shot up by 5,455 percent, increasing to $750 per pill. Turing's CEO, Martin Shkreli, was labeled by many as the most hated man in America.

There are plenty of other examples of greed, of medications being overpriced for profit, such as cycloserine and doxycycline, but this is not the standard model. Drug companies provide cures and alleviate suffering, but they also have to make a profit to stay afloat. The availability of generic medications is perhaps a lifesaver for many patients, costing far less than brand-name drugs such as Daraprim. The generic form of Prozac is cheap, just $4 for a 30-day supply. The major expense remains finding a provider, being evaluated, and receiving the prescription.

The Diagnostic and Statistical Manual of Mental Disorders

The rise of Prozac, perhaps, would not have been as successful had there not been a reliable way to categorize depression and understand its symptoms, which the *Diagnostic and Statistical Manual of Mental Disorders (DSM)* does in great detail. Now in its fifth edition, the expansive manual has come a long way from its slim first edition in 1952, which did not even use the term depression, the closest match being "manic depressive reaction, depressive type" [53]. The manual is now in its fifth edition and is anything but slim.

Psychiatry is often seen as a century behind other medical specialties, primarily because of a lag in applying empirical research. According to Nassir Ghaemi, psychiatry has been playing catch-up and "sits in the same place scientifically as medicine did at the end of the nineteenth century" [7]. Although a critic of the *DSM*, van Praag admits that when he began his residency in 1960, "research, that is to say, empirical research, was virtually nonexistent in psychiatry" [59]. He goes further, recognizing the need for a clear way to diagnose patients: "Diagnoses were often incomplete, not standardized, and not based on operationalized criteria. The result was a confusion of tongues that seriously detracted from psychiatry's scientific credibility" [59].

A major reason for this lack of empirical precision and scientific credibility was the binding of psychiatry to psychoanalysis, which emphasized the unconscious mind versus the brain. It was a decline in psychoanalysis and the rise of biological psychiatry that fueled this need to catch up empirically. According to Shorter, "in the vacuum created by the discarding of psychoanalysis, confusion reigned as to how best go about therapy" [18]. But the battle of psychiatry to attain its rightful status within medicine was not easy. Says Shorter, "In the 1950s and early 1960s, psychoanalysis consolidated its hold over American psychiatry" [18]. In 1968, the *DSM-II* was published, and "six of the ten members of the drafting committee were analysts or belonged to sympathetic organizations" [18].

However, it was in the 1960s that psychoanalysis began to lose its grip over psychiatry, and psychiatry's concern became getting the diagnosis right "on the basis of presenting symptoms, then conducting a proper investigation to come up with a clinical diagnosis..." [18]. The *DSM-II* provided little guidance and was curious in many ways. For example, the *DSM-II* came under pressure from gays, who demanded that homosexuality be removed as a diagnosis. The *DSM-II* had much to say about "chronic brain syndrome" but had little to say about depression, other than it could be a component of manic-depressive illness and was categorized, as many other disorders, as a "reaction" (a holdover from psychoanalysis) in the form of a neurosis [97]. These factors, along with insurers' desire for more precise diagnoses, led to a revamp of the *DSM*, with the third edition released in 1980 [18]. The physicians in charge of producing the *DSM-III* recognized a move away from psychoanalysis toward biological psychiatry and "a redirection of the discipline toward a scientific course" [18].

Depression Since Prozac—Finding the True Self

The manual went from a psychoanalytically influenced referential diagnostic tool to an objective, criteria-based system that linked measurable symptoms with specific mental disorders such as depression [98]. The much-improved and voluminous *DSM-III* was an important move in clinical practice to overcome the antipsychiatry movement, as epitomized by the famous Rosenhan Experiment, published in *Science* under the title "On Being Sane in Insane Places" [99]. Rosenhan sent healthy subjects to various mental hospitals in several states and had them fake auditory hallucinations. Each "fake patient" was diagnosed with a mental disorder and hospitalized, and all were later released, having recanted the auditory hallucinations, but usually with a diagnosis of schizophrenia [99]. This was "fake illness" much as we have "fake news" today, and bolstered those opposed to psychiatry, most famously the Scientologists and Thomas Szasz.

In the *DSM-III*, homosexuality was removed as a disease of sexual deviance, and a great leap forward was made in terms of providing clinicians with a tool to differentially diagnose a particular mental illness, enhancing psychiatry's reputation as a "respected scientific discipline" [32]. The "*DSM-III* listed 265 different disorders, up one-third from the 180 in *DSM-II*" [18] and "adopted the principle of multiaxial diagnosis…a compromise of a diversity of expert opinions" [59]. Great strides were made in classifying depression as a specific disorder. Instead of referring to depression as a reactive neurosis, the term "major depression" was created. To represent a less severe form of depression that was persistent, the term "dysthymic disorder" was introduced. Good news for psychiatrists was that they not only had a clear way to diagnose depression, but also there were antidepressants and therapy to treat it. This, of course, raises some criticism. Ghaemi observes that having these new classifications gave "psychotherapists something to bill" [7], but he also observes that with the *DSM-III*, "American psychiatry moved from pure psychoanalytic ideology to at least some science" [7].

The *DSM-IV*, published in 1994, "came in with 297 disorders" [18], and this expansion in sheer numbers continued with the *DSM-V*, published in 2013. The evolution of the manual sought to affirm and expand research-based nosology (the science of diagnosing). According to the *DSM-V*, the manual is "intended to serve as a practical, functional, and flexible guide for organizing information that can aid in the accurate diagnosis and treatment of mental disorders" [100]. The authors recognized that "mental disorders do not always fit completely within the boundaries of a single disorder," [100] which some think keeps it at a distance from "real medicine" where specific diagnoses and syndromes have more concrete definitions. Says van Praag, "In day-to-day practice I rarely saw textbook cases; instead patients usually showed (parts of) several syndromes" [59]. This overlapping of disorders, of course, is something for the trained and astute psychiatrist or psychologist to differentiate. It is very often the case that multiple diagnoses are given to patients, and not just one.

The *DSM* still has its critics. "Why so many diagnoses?" is a common question. This seems to accuse psychiatry of wanting as many diagnoses as possible for which to bill. According to Dan Blazer,

> Psychiatrists should not attempt to name everything. In our investigative studies, we should abandon the assumption that there is a specific, widespread disease 'major depression' that captures the vast majority of people experiencing disabling, depressive symptoms. [57]

This argument does not seem to help those who are living with depression. Admitting your depression places you in a box with a label, but that is where healing can begin. It is always most important to remember the patient's best interest, and patients feel more secure knowing the specific problem they are facing. Even if the depression lifts, one is still vulnerable. A similar situation is the alcoholic who is taught that they will always be an alcoholic, the idea being that that a diagnosis keeps the patient aware. Holly Lynn Ryan brings up psychiatry heretic Thomas Szasz, who wrote *The Myth of Mental Illness.* Szasz is famous for saying, "In the past, men created witches: now they create mental patients" [101].

Despite admitting that psychiatrists in the 1950s and 60s were in a muddle regarding diagnoses, van Praag is critical of the *DSM*. He notes that in his early days, there were only two types of depression: endogenous (vital) and neurotic (personal). Speaking in 1993 when the *DSM-IV* was available, he says, "Today's classification of the major psychiatric disorders is as confusing as it used to be some 30 years ago" but that now "the chaos is codified" and based solely on expert opinion [59]. Expert opinion is a good thing, though, and codifying what is admittedly confusing seems to be a logical step to take. It is not easy to definitively diagnose a person with mental illness, but the *DSM* assists that process. Affronted by biological psychiatry, van Praag is worried about the medicalization of psychiatry, which plays down the "psychological and social aspects of abnormal behavior" [59]. Although the *DSM* is now research-based, van Praag sees the disorders as "largely the products of our own making" [59]. But if researchers discover a particular disease, then it is their job to define it in such a way that it can be reliably diagnosed. This is good for the patient. There isn't just one type of cancer; there are more than a hundred. But still, van Praag says, "Psychiatry has little to gain from hierarchical diagnostic systems and much to lose…" [59].

Concrete examples of disorders that seemed to flower overnight include social phobias and multiple personality disorder.

According to Elliott, the number of articles on social phobia went from 17 (1967–1983) to 1,137 in 1998. The *DSM-III* took notice and incorporated this "new" disorder into its pages [39]. Multiple personality disorder (MPD) became an official diagnosis of the American Psychiatric Association in 1980. Ten years later, there were hundreds of cases of MPD, whereas previously it had been a mere curiosity [49]. Says Ian Hacking, "How can a mental disorder be so at the whim of place and time" [49]? One has to consider other factors, such as doctors' education in diagnosing the illness and popular media, which often latch onto a disorder, as with *Sybil: The Classic True Story of a Woman Possessed by Sixteen Personalities,* first published in 1973. With depression, much popular literature has brought the disorder into the mainstream, which is a good thing. Ultimately, it is about the patient. Says Hacking, "Knowledge of causes helps us prevent illness. But causation also matters to theory. When we know the causes, we feel confident that we have identified a disease entity, something more than a cluster of symptoms" [49].

Prozac Today

According to a Mental Health America report (2018), 16 million U.S. citizens live with major depression [102]. Barber notes that "the SSRIs have been proven to have real efficacy for many if not most people who suffer from major depression" [22]. Regarding mild depression, he states that "there is no evidence or only very limited evidence that they work for people with 'subsyndromal' depression" [22]. This is up for debate, but the SSRIs do work well for those with major depression, and if serotonin is the key to taking the edge off of depression then it should work just as well for the mildly depressed or those suffering from chronic forms of depression, dysthymic disorder, and other disorders that are "subsyndromal" for the six major symptoms of major depression.

Depression Since Prozac—Finding the True Self

Suffering from depression, whether mild or severe, one should have the opportunity to be relieved of its symptoms.

In general, the news is good for those with depression. There are more medication options for treatment than ever before, and at reasonable prices if one uses generic forms. The fever has pitched, and Prozac is here to stay, riding on its merits rather quietly today versus the outbursts of the 1990s and early 2000s. Says Kramer, a fan of Prozac, "Prozac enjoyed the career of the true celebrity—renown, followed by rumors, then notoriety, scandal, and lawsuits, and finally a quiet rehabilitation" [23]. Criticized by many, Kramer, a clinical psychiatrist, is a rational advocate for the SSRIs as well as behavioral therapy. But even he is cautious:

> When faced with a medication that does transform, even in this friendly way, I became aware of my own irrational discomfort, my sense that for a drug to have such a pronounced effect is inherently unnatural, unsafe, uncanny [23].

Uncanny is a great word with which Prozac beneficiaries, and writers Elizabeth Wurtzel (*Prozac Nation*) and Lauren Slater (*Prozac Diaries*) would agree. Says Susan Squier of Slater, "Prozac has opened her up to the beauty of life in the moment…" [103]. Lifted from a deep depression, one has to wonder how it can be so easy to overcome an illness that kills, an illness that is the number one cause of disability worldwide. Whether for or against Prozac, "every article on Prozac has this caveat…: for the person with serious clinical depression, antidepressant medications are a lifesaving medical intervention" [48]. Most important is how Prozac has changed the way we view depression. We now see depression as an illness that is real and that responds well to treatment with minimal side effects. Shorter notes that "the Prozac episode produced one massive benefit for the public good:

It helped psychiatric conditions begin to seem acceptable in the destigmatization of mental illness" [18]. The battle to destigmatize mental illness in general, of course, is not over, but well on its way concerning depression.

One final note: Roughly half of all persons diagnosed with depression do not receive treatment [104]. How many people who are undiagnosed is unknown. Causes for not seeking treatment vary, including stigma and inability to afford the medications or therapy. The National Center for Health Statistics (NCHS) estimates that in 2015, 10.6 percent of Americans were uninsured, in addition to those unable to obtain treatment [90]. It is vital that those not receiving treatment be given the opportunity that the treated have. Again, as Wurtzel said so well, depression "ruins... lives," and that need not be the case [27].

From the discovery of the first neurotransmitter, acetylcholine, in the 1920s to the first antidepressants in the 1950s, Prozac spent 16 years in development before it was released in 1987. Since then, office visits for depression and prescriptions for antidepressants have soared, but still, not everyone is being reached. Depression, as with cancer and heart disease, deserves every effort to stem its tide of despair, including effective medications such as Prozac.

Prozac Under Fire

Under fire from all sides since 1987, Prozac has endured its critics and become a household name, rendering depression into a palatable disease over which one no longer has to whisper. But we do not have to look far to see the battle being waged against Prozac and medications like it: Say P.C. Gøtzsche, A.H. Young, and J. Crace, "Psychiatric drugs are responsible for the deaths of more than half a million people aged 65 and older each year in the Western world..." [105]. That's quite hard to fathom and does not, of course, take into consideration those whose lives were saved or made tolerable. According to them, we could "stop almost all psychotropic drug use without deleterious effect..." [105]. This statement is in the context of clinical trials and their designs, which "underplay harms and overplay benefits" [105]. The clinical trials approving Prozac and other antidepressants have caused quite a bit of controversy, some finding that Prozac works no better than placebo [106]. It is true that the initial phases of clinical trials with Prozac seemed to show that Prozac did not work, but the study population being used was found to be loaded with patients with severe and intractable depression, and a more viable selection of patients showed that Prozac worked. Entering studies with exaggerated depression scores means that the patient is bound to get better on placebo since there is so much room to improve, giving the placebo effect credence [23].

The Placebo Effect

This battle of placebo versus Prozac ranges far and wide. Prozac enthusiast Peter Kramer notes that "the placebo is a pale doppelganger, taking the form of the active intervention but lacking the enlivening element...It is there to be thrown away" [23]. What he means is that the result being sought lies with the treatment versus the placebo, and an effective drug will allow you to discard the placebo as meaningless. The placebo effect works because the patient thinks he must be getting better simply because he is being treated. Many say that Prozac works because of the placebo effect. People think they are supposed to get better, and so they do. But faking not being depressed is a challenging task. Somewhat balanced in their approach, Irving Kirsch and Guy Saperstein say, "Our results are in agreement with those of other meta-analyses in revealing a substantial placebo effect in antidepressant medication and also a considerable benefit of medication over placebo." [107]

Gøtzsche et al. accuse trials of being biased toward favoring medications since the patients were already on other psychiatric medications, which they had to stop before the trial. This left them vulnerable and in need of improvement. They say, "This design exaggerates the benefits of treatment and increases the harms in the placebo group, and it has driven patients taking placebo to suicide in trials in schizophrenia" [105]. This is certainly a worry, but it could also be that the medications previously taken were not working, leaving more room for improvement.

Kirsch and Saperstein affirm many times, based on their meta-analysis of clinical trials, that Prozac works no better than placebo, saying that "for a typical patient, 75 percent of the benefit obtained from the active drug would also have been obtained from an inactive placebo" [107]. Says Kramer, "Kirsch's conclusions proved influential. It became commonplace for popular writing to suggest that antidepressants do not work at all" [23]. Although Kramer and others would disagree, "placebo effects are produced by specific response expectancies and...they cannot be fully explained by other factors such as classical conditioning, therapeutic relationship, or more general expectancies for improvement" [107]. Kramer, from his personal experience with trial subjects, says,

> In 'candidate drug trials,' as the research on new medicines is called, contact with raters [those who are assessing the depression of the placebo and treatment groups] is extensive and supportive, so placebo response rates run high. The patients who sign on rarely resemble the depressed patients I have seen, now or in my training. [23]

And there are other arguments for the alleged placebo effects of Prozac, including the miracle of "spontaneous remission" or "life changes, the passage of time, or other factors" [107]. There is the argument that patients guess when they have been given the placebo or the drug and respond accordingly. Someone receiving the placebo may mistakenly think they are receiving the Prozac and imagine that they are feeling better, a placebo effect. This, of course, is not desired as it skews the results, showing that the placebo is as effective or more effective than the drug.

Kramer, too, is critical of clinical trials, which are imperfect for many reasons. Regarding Food and Drug Administration (FDA) trials, he says, "[T]he trials are a lousy source of information about antidepressant efficacy, and it is shocking that an important medical question…has been debated using them as a reflection of reality" [23].

He cites another bias introduced by trials. Often, it is the poor who are selected because they have the time and need the remuneration. Kramer notes that participating in a trial for someone marginalized alters their world temporarily:

> For the duration of a trial, participants enjoy higher income, richer social contacts, attention from doctors and nurses, access to transportation, time in an attractive

setting, structured days, and a sense of purpose...Even on placebo, these patients ought to get better. [23]

Another problem is rater bias. Patients may try to guess which arm of the study they are in, but the raters, who are blinded to who is in which group, often themselves guess which group is which and may, through their actions, influence the patient.

Also, as Kramer notes, just the very fact that all patients know that there is a placebo arm and think that maybe they have gotten the placebo when they have not impedes a true measurement within the treatment group. If a participant thinks that a placebo is being used, then "drug effects reported in controlled trials may be lower than real inherent drug effects enjoyed by patients treated through their doctor's prescribing" [23]. This is often referred to as the lessebo effect. However, Kramer wants us to look at the clinical improvements he sees in his patients, such as Tess, in his book *Listening to Prozac*: "The Tess that she had been on Prozac now seemed to her the true Tess" [40]. One scenario that the placebo fails to elicit is "improvement at three weeks followed by continued well-being at every subsequent point of observation" [23].

Another criticism of antidepressants is that they only work for the severely depressed and that those with mild to moderate depression benefit less. Kramer calls this the "severity hypothesis," saying that "it dates to the earliest days of the psychopharmacologic era, when lesser depression was psychotherapy's domain" [23]. Kramer also warns of the "floor effect," which means that with mild depression, there is little room to improve, and the resulting shift is more likely to be static [23]. This results in an underestimation "of the efficacy in the treatment of less ill patients" [23]. In other words, treating a serious case of depression has the potential to yield greater results as the floor is so far away.

Continuing, grievously at times, to register his discontent with the authority placed in clinical trials, Kramer points to an aspect of bias in recruiting called baseline score inflation. When a rater is recruiting patients for a trial, she may be tempted to bump a borderline case to the minimal score needed to participate to increase enrollment [23]. This gives less room for improvement. A last critique of clinical trials is what Kramer calls the differential sieve. In the placebo arm of a trial, it is the healthy who survive the trial. This yields an improvement in the placebo group compared with sicker people in the treatment group, making it appear that the placebo is working wonders. Ultimately, Kramer wants us to look upon clinical trial data with a discerning eye and says emphatically, "Placebos don't prevent depression, and antidepressants do" [23].

Thus, the placebo effect, it seems, is a red herring that draws attention away from the real benefits of Prozac and medications like it. It appears that Prozac works best with serious depression, but that is because the seriously depressed have more room to improve. Those with any form of depression deserve the right to feel better.

Antidepressants and Children and Teenagers

The use of antidepressants in children and teenagers is controversial. The idea of medicating our youth raises ire and needed caution, but as always, the benefits must be weighed against the risks. Mary Leonard notes that

> there are legitimate concerns that Prozac and its sisters Zoloft, Paxil, Effexor and Serzone—so easy to get, too quick a fix—might be overused just as Ritalin has been for hyperactivity. Prozac will make it easy to prescribe mellowing antidepressants to children who simply may be acting

like children. [94]

However, according to Mental Health America (2018), "11.93 percent of youth (age 12-17) report suffering from at least one major depressive episode (MDE) in the past" and "8.2 percent of youth (or 1.9 million youth) experienced severe depression" [102], somewhat mirroring adult depression prevalence. Says Charles Barber, a critic of antidepressants in general, "For so many kids today, the taking of a psychiatric drug is simply part of growing up, no big deal, one of the way stations of youth..." [22]. In 2000, Joseph Glenmullen noted that "half a million children are prescribed the drugs..." [25]. In the U.S., a drug company survey "found that between 1995 and 1999 use of Prozac-like drugs for children aged 7–12 increased by 151 percent, and in those aged under 6 by 580 percent" [17]. Many seem amazed that we are treating our children with Prozac and similar medications. Leonard reported in *The Boston Globe* that "It is no joke" [94] that Prozac (or rather its generic form fluoxetine) was becoming available in a liquid oral form with a mint flavor, manufactured by OSG Norwich Pharmaceutical [108].

After approving Prozac for adults, it took the FDA an additional six years to approve Prozac for children and teens. In 2003, the FDA approved Prozac to treat children and adolescents "ages 7 to 17 for depression and obsessive-compulsive disorder (OCD)" [109]. According to the CDC, "When children feel persistent sadness and hopelessness, they may be diagnosed with depression" [110]. The CDC adds that "for youth ages 10-24 years, suicide is the leading form of death" [110]. It is interesting that when discussing treatment, the CDC does not mention medication as an option but instead focuses on cognitive behavioral therapy, nutritious food, physical activity, and sufficient sleep, all of which are important but which may not be sufficient [110]. Other an-

Depression Since Prozac—Finding the True Self

tidepressants, such as the tricyclic antidepressants, have been approved for use in children, specifically imipramine, which has also been used to ward off bedwetting.

The potential for suicidal thoughts and behavior among youth as a result of taking Prozac has caused warranted concern. In October 2004, the FDA

> directed manufacturers of all antidepressant drugs to revise the labeling for their products to include a boxed warning and expanded warning statements that alert health care providers to an increased risk of suicidality (suicidal thinking and behavior) in children and adolescents being treated with these agents. [111]

In 2006, an advisory committee to the FDA recommended that the agency extend the warning to young adults up to age 25. The prescription insert for Prozac and other antidepressants contains the black box warning, which reads "Increased risk of suicidal thinking and behavior in children, adolescents, and young adults taking antidepressants" [15]. Other antidepressant classes also include this warning, not just Prozac and the SSRIs. In an FDA review in 2004, "no completed suicides occurred among nearly 2,200 children treated with SSRI medications," but "about 4 percent of those taking SSRI medications experienced suicidal thinking or behavior, including actual suicide attempts—twice the rate of those taking placebo, or sugar pills" [15]. This is what led to the black box warning for Prozac and a specific list of other antidepressants.

Another SSRI, Paxil (paroxetine), was singled out by critics and scientists. In 2001, the maker of Paxil, GlaxoSmithKline (GSK), formerly SmithKline Beecham, published the infamous "Study 329," stating that their analysis did "support that paroxetine is beneficial in treating adolescents with major depression"

[112]. Following the report, "Prescriptions of antidepressants to young people surged, increasing by 36 percent between 2002 and 2003...The growth slowed after regulators ordered the black-box warnings on labels" [113]. But researchers long doubted the claims of Paxil's efficacy and desired to reexamine the data. In 2012, GSK agreed to pay $3 billion in a fraud settlement with the United States government [114]. In 2015, the *British Medical Journal* reached the opposite conclusion of Study 329 using GSK's original data, finding that "Neither paroxetine nor high dose imipramine showed efficacy for major depression in adolescents, and there was an increase in harms with both drugs" [115]. However, "The maker of Paxil...said it stood by the original conclusions" [113].

Despite the *British Medical Journal* study, antidepressants do work in children and teenagers. According to the NIMH,

> Certain antidepressant medications, called selective serotonin reuptake inhibitors (SSRIs), can be beneficial to children and adolescents with MDD [major depressive disorder]. Certain types of psychological therapies also have been shown to be effective. [15]

But the rhetoric against treating children and teens is still strong. According to the Citizens Commission on Human Rights (CCHR) website,

> When psychiatrists or doctors prescribe dangerous, potentially life-threatening psychiatric drugs to children without the parent or legal guardian's consent, they should be charged with reckless endangerment and/or child endangerment because these drugs are documented to cause side effects including, but not limited to, suicide, mania, heart problems, stroke, diabetes, death and sudden death. [88]

A major controversy is the screening of children for depression, which began in 2002, according to Julian Whitaker, who is with CCHR. He cites a now-defunct group called Teen Screen, which aimed to "'expand early detection of mental illness by mainstreaming evidence-based mental health checkups as a routine procedure in adolescent health care, schools, and other youth-serving settings'" [106]. But, screening for a debilitating illness such as depression is a good idea, given depression's prevalence and consequences, but Whitaker makes it clear that he thinks screening for depression is out of line.

> You should under no circumstances allow your children to participate in school-based mental health screenings. Do not be mislead [sic] by doublespeak from school boards, psychiatrists, counselors, or teachers. Despite their veneer of identifying and helping those at risk, mental health screenings are little more than fishing expeditions, casting a broad net and reeling in millions of new psychiatric drug users. [106]

So, the battle is neither won nor lost, and the issue of treating children with "adult" medications will remain controversial.

Prozac and Violence

Prozac has been cited as a link to violence in both popular and medical literature. From *The Sun,* the British tabloid, we have this headline: "Axe for top cop turned into bully by Prozac" [79]. From Anna Moore, we learn that "after six days on Prozac, Patricia Williamson, 60, killed herself in her bath in Texas while her husband ate breakfast downstairs" [17]. Further, "anecdotal evidence in the popular press has suggested that use of SSRIs is linked with outbursts of anger and aggression and with suicide" [79]. One of the most famous cases of Prozac associated with violence is that of Joseph Wesbecker in 1989. He had been on Prozac for less than a month when he shot and killed eight employees at Standard Gravure in Louisville, Kentucky. He then killed himself [17].

So, does Prozac induce violence toward others and the self? M.T. Walsh and T.G. Dinan report that "no increased susceptibility to aggression or suicidality can be connected with fluoxetine or any other SSRI" [79]. They cite the lack of credible evidence and consider the nature of the SSRIs:

> It would seem likely that enhancement of serotonergic function, for example by prescription of appropriate SSRI medication in a manner suitable to individual patients, might be reasonably expected to have a beneficial effect on aggression and suicidality. [79]

From their own review of available evidence, Walsh and Dinan note "anger attacks disappeared in the majority (between 64 and 84 percent) of patients who reported them prior to taking fluoxetine [Prozac]" [79]. In 1991, the FDA weighed in on Prozac's safety and "exonerated the drug," a panel finding that there was no credible evidence "that Prozac caused suicidal or violent impulses" [25].

Mention of suicidality and the SSRIs requires a look at the Teicher Report. In M.H. Teicher et al.'s article, "Emergence of intense suicidal preoccupation during fluoxetine treatment," they created notable alarm with stories of "six depressed patients free of recent serious suicidal ideation [who] developed intense, violent suicidal preoccupation after 2-7 weeks of fluoxetine [Prozac] treatment" [116]. Much sensational press and criticism of the report were generated. Researchers carefully asked how a drug that increases serotonin could cause suicidal ideation "because there is considerable evidence of serotonin deficiency in patients who attempt or complete suicide...and fluoxetine selectively enhances serotonergic transmission" [117]. The Teicher Report, though debunked, remains influential.

A 2000 study by Donovan et al. found that patients taking Prozac had the highest relative risk of suicidal behavior, 6.6, versus those taking amitriptyline; that is, patients were 6.6 times more likely to engage in deliberate self-harm (DSH) than persons taking the older drug [118]. The authors noted, however, that medications such as Prozac are safer in overdose versus the TCAs, such as amitriptyline [118]. They do concede, though, saying that "it is difficult to attribute the cause of DSH behaviour to antidepressant treatment when such behaviour can also occur spontaneously during the course of depressive illness" [118].

In 2004, the FDA issued the black-box warning for the SSRIs, warning of "an increased risk of suicidal thinking, feeling, and behavior in young people" [119]. The move was predicated on data that showed a 2 percent risk of suicide with placebo versus 4 percent with an antidepressant [119]. Many in the medical community were concerned over this move, worried that it would prevent those in need of treatment from seeking it or receiving it. Researchers followed up on this concern, finding "significant reductions in antidepressant use within 2 years after the FDA advisory was issued: relative reductions of 31.0 percent, 24.3 percent, and 14.5 percent among adolescents, young adults, and adults, respectively" [119]. The warning was revised in 2007, stating,

> Depression and certain other psychiatric disorders are themselves associated with increases in the risk of suicide. Patients of all ages who are started on antidepressant therapy should be monitored appropriately and observed closely for clinical worsening, suicidality, or unusual changes in behavior. [120]

Between 2003 and 2005, "the proportion of adults with depression who did not receive an antidepressant increased from 20 percent to 30 percent during the same period" [119]. Friedman concluded that "it is certainly plausible that the declines in depression diagnoses and antidepressant prescriptions might reflect the attitudes of both patients and physicians in the face of the controversy over, and media coverage of, the FDA advisory" [119]. The warning could have discouraged medication and made more people vulnerable to suicide. Thus, did the warning actually cause more harm than good?

Prozac and medications like it have been tried by the fire of society as well as methodical research. The good news is that Prozac has been under the microscope and proven a worthy treatment for depressive disorders and other diseases such as bulimia, obsessive-compulsive disorder, and panic disorder. Never before has a single drug elicited the outpouring of public and scientific attention that Prozac has received. Many other medications have fallen under scrutiny, such as Valium and Ritalin, but Prozac remains the measure of society's fascination with mental illness and its treatment, and it works.

Marketing Antidepressants

Developing a new medication, conducting clinical trials, and introducing it to the world is expensive. What matters is that those who need it to function receive it. Drug companies, of course, want to make as much profit as possible, and that can be a real conflict, especially if the drug is not affordable. As Kimberly Emmons notes, "People with a depressive illness cannot merely 'pull themselves together' and get better" [56]. They need help, often in the form of medication. In general, a patent on a new medication lasts for twenty years, and then the generic manufacturers can jump in and take their share of the market. There are also additional terms of exclusivity, which last up to seven years.

What makes Prozac a marketing dream is well said by David Wong et al.:

> The introduction of fluoxetine, which was the first SSRI to be marketed in the United States, has arguably had a pronounced effect on the treatment of depression, on depressed patients and on the perception of mental illness; its introduction has been said to have ushered in a new era of safe and effective pharmacotherapy for depression...The sustained effectiveness of fluoxetine, low side-effect profile, overdose safety, once-a-day dosing, lack of a requirement for dose titration and improved risk-benefit ratio have led to widespread use by physicians. [66]

Of course, drug companies such as Eli Lilly, the maker of Prozac, are experts in the marketing arena and understand human behavior. According to Holly Ryan, whose PhD dissertation is a valuable resource regarding direct-to-consumer (DTC) advertising of antidepressants, "Emotional health is not a stable, fixed entity; it is a rhetorically constructed concept that, in recent years, the pharmaceutical companies have been a persuasive and pervasive force in developing" [32]. Although depression is a disease versus a simple issue of emotional health, the drug companies realize that to appeal to a wider audience, it is best to pitch the drug as widely as possible, thus the label "emotional health." Ryan, a drug-company skeptic, further says, "Everyday emotions such as sadness, loneliness, and apathy are medicalized into illness, and this produces a medical discourse around depression" [32]. She is right, of course, but depression as an entity is a disease, an illness, and much clinical and laboratory research has affirmed depression as a legitimate "thing." And once you have the illness, the medications will hopefully follow, being prescribed if you need them. Says Carl Elliott, "The market moves to fill a demand for happiness as efficiently as it moves to fill a demand for spark plugs or home computers" [39]. Although jaded in tone, Elliott is right in the sense that once a market is recognized, it receives the full attention of those able to supply it.

In 1906, the Pure Food and Drugs Act was signed into law, marking the first time that some federal oversight was given to regulate the marketing of medications. The first regulation that addressed advertising was the Federal Food, Drug, and Cosmetic Act of 1938, which "restricted the advertisement of prescription drugs in the United States to medical journals and other professional publications" [32]. Thus, advertising circumvented the general population, and it was up to doctors to get the word out. This was an effort to "protect consumers from making uninformed healthcare choices" [32]. It was in 1962 that "Congress specifically granted the FDA statutory authority to regulate prescription drug labeling and advertising" [121], leading to DTC advertising.

In 1983, after reviewing drug company DTC advertising, the federal government suspended DTC advertising, but in 1985, the Food and Drug Administration (FDA) withdrew the short-lived moratorium, stating that "current regulations governing prescription drug advertising provide sufficient safeguards to protect consumers" [32]. According to C. Lee Ventola, "This ruling triggered an onslaught of widespread print, but not broadcast DTC advertising" [121]. In addition to a relaxation of the rules, "there was a cultural shift [that] occurred that caused patients to start actively participating in medical decision-making with their health care providers" [121]. Drug companies now had doctors to disseminate the medications, as well as an informed public seeking the medicines. The favoring of print ads over broadcast was a matter of cost. Drug company DTC advertising had to meet the requirements of "fair balance" and "brief summary," something that small print was amenable to but not feasible for a TV ad at the time. In terms of possible impact, "The share of psychiatric patients receiving prescriptions increased from a quarter of all office visits in 1975 to fully one-half by 1990" [18]. Informing consumers generally leads to increased prescriptions.

A further relaxation of the rules on DTC advertising in the United States occurred in 1997. According to the National Institute for Health Care Management (NIHCM), this relaxing of rules "sparked the...rapid growth in the mass media marketing of prescription drugs...The action made it easier for companies to launch TV, print, and radio ad campaigns" [122], opening a direct pipeline to prescription-drug consumers.

Ryan refers to the drug companies' marketing campaigns as a "a technology of normalization" [32]. What must be done is take an illness such as depression, identify it as abnormal, and then present the way "by which the abnormal can be subjected to reform through techniques of the self—specifically the act of confession" [32]. One has to recognize and admit that one is depressed and that a viable solution exists. Referring to print ads for antidepressants, Emmons recognizes a "broadest possible audience" that is being reached by dumbing down the clinical aspects of depression into softer terminology such as "'restlessness' or 'difficulty concentrating' as symptoms that demand treatment" [56]. The drug companies are pitching a product based in science, defining what is abnormal in layperson's terms, but with a clear rhetorical strategy geared toward consumption. In 2004, the FDA again revised regulations concerning DTC advertising, eliminating the need to reprint complete prescribing information in print product claim ads and allowing the inclusion of a "simplified brief summary" instead [121].

A major criticism of DTC advertising is summed up by Elliott: "[T]he industry has learned that the key to selling psychiatric drugs is to sell the illnesses they treat" [39]. Companies use clever slogans aimed at the educated consumer's desire to normalize: Prozac: Welcome back; Paxil: Your life is waiting; Wellbutrin: I'm ready to experience life; Effexor: The change you deserve. The disease is reduced to simple terms with an obvious solution: the medication. The consumer understands that to regain normalcy, action is necessary. Those not seeking the norm become "marginalized" [32]. Ryan adds, "These ads are not simply selling drugs; they are selling a way of life, a normative framework for which to view and behave in the world" [32]. This normative framework, with its specific language, is, according to Ian Hacking, a "semantic contagion" that causes the public to identify with a disorder, enabling it to spread [39]. Barbara Heifferon and Stuart C. Brown note the significance of this seemingly simple spread of language specific to depression: "Language events within the medical professions are often literally life and death rhetorical situations that create an even greater need to bring the power of in situ language study to bear" [123].

Advertisements work these feelings of sadness and loneliness into the abnormal. It is not normal to feel this way, say the ads, and the ads provide a solution such as Prozac. The ads "provide a modifying activity that will help people become more normal: taking prescription medication" [32]. Ryan identifies six stages to normalization engineered by the ads: (1) Establish the norm, (2) Identify with the abnormal, (3) Confess to abnormality, (4) Seek ways to become normal, (5) Become persuaded by practices to become normal, and (6) Engage in behaviors that promote the normal [32]. By conceding one's depression through a series of logical steps, one first becomes abnormal and then, once treated, normalized. The ads have great power in encouraging people with the symptoms of depression to seek treatment. Ryan sees this mainly as an end to profit, but how else would one advertise?

Being depressed and recognizing the need for treatment, whether through insight or ads, does not matter in the end. There is, of course, the chance that someone without depression may become convinced by the ads that they are depressed, but a visit to a keen clinician should result in nontreatment. Distrustful, though, Elliott warns that for doctors "the body and mind are objects of control" [39]. According to him, doctors desire to control a patient as "objects of therapeutic control, a human life becomes a project that can be tweaked and reworked and adjusted in accordance with a person's own private wishes and desires." [39]

Thus, a person convinced they are depressed in the hands of a self-interested doctor may wind up under treatment. Having seen the ad, the patient may tell their doctor about a specific medication that they think they need. According to D.L. Rosenthal et al., "A survey found that 71 percent of family physicians believe that direct-to-consumer advertising pressures physicians into prescribing drugs that they would not ordinarily prescribe"

[124]. But, is it worse to have the occasional case of unnecessary treatment, a false positive, versus truly ill patients being passed by? Rosenthal et al., though, add, "Relatively few people surveyed (less than 6 percent), however, actually received a prescription for the advertised drug after being prompted by direct-to-consumer advertising to ask their doctor about the drug" [124].

One factor that must not be forgotten is that Prozac has made it okay to be depressed. The widespread attention it has received has given depression household status. It is no longer shameful to be depressed and okay to seek treatment, although bias still exists. A criticism is that the ads have fostered a drug-seeking culture [32]. Has not our culture always been a drug-seeking culture? From patent medicines of the nineteenth century to amphetamine use in the first half of the twentieth century to more modern medications such as Valium, people have always sought medications to make themselves feel better. DTC advertising certainly adds a layer of complexity, and the drug companies cannot help but appear complicit in this drug-seeking behavior. However, no one, except perhaps the hypochondriac or person suffering from Munchausen syndrome, desires to be depressed. Ryan observes, "I argue that the current psychiatric and scientific discourses of depression lay the foundation for the pharmaceutical companies to aggressively market antidepressants" [32]. Certainly, the drug companies are pitching the net widely, using terms such as sad, empty, or hopeless that may exaggerate the popular confines of true depression, but these are terms used in the DSM that clinically differentiate depression from normalcy [100]. Nothing is being made up or intentionally exaggerated.

Indeed, the ads are slick and effective, but that is the nature of advertising. Ryan mentions an ad for Zoloft: "Do you feel sad or lonely? These are common signs of depression." Ryan admits that the advertisers are not lying, that these are indeed clinical signs of depression. She rightly notes that "to be diagnosed as depressed, these emotions must be persistent, severe, and unusual for the individual. Without qualifying these emotions, the pharmaceutical companies have taken common human emotions and given them pathology" [32]. There is certainly room for DTC ads to be more exacting, but as long as those in need are being positively impacted, we should be thankful. Consider an ad featuring a slick kayak with a smiling paddler in the middle of a whitewater rapid. The consumer gets excited and buys a kayak only to find that getting the kayak to the creek and then having a scary experience in a rapid causes him to lose interest. In fact, kayaking is the number one outdoor sport where people try it once and give it up. Should we blame the kayak manufacturer for the purchase?

According to Alan Gross, "rhetoric is more than window-dressing; it concerns the necessary and sufficient conditions for the creation of persuasive discourse in any field. Science cannot be excluded by fiat" [125]. Prescription medications represent scientific endeavors, and the science and art of marketing those medications depend on the same mechanisms as marketing a kayak or a car. Science is "a rhetorical enterprise, centered on persuasion" [125]. It follows that the science of marketing is also centered on persuasion. Healthcare and medications are not an exception to the rule. Pharmaceutical companies need to sell their medications and rely on the tried-and-true methods that work, just as any industry does. This may at times come across as overly aggressive, but still, roughly half of depressed patients remain untreated. As stated earlier, "Every 40 seconds a person dies by suicide somewhere in the world and many more attempt suicide" [10]. In the United States, according to the CDC, suicide is the second leading cause of death among persons aged 15-24 years, the second among persons aged 25-34 years, the fourth among persons aged 35-54 years…" [8]. Suicide rates have not decreased with the introduction of the SSRIs and could possibly be higher without them. The danger of creating a false positive for depression has to be weighed against the desperate need to help those in need.

Still, critics abound: "Prozac made it acceptable for drugs to be, simply and solely, lifestyle agents…" [22]. What about sadness and grief as a lifestyle? What is the use of that? Prozac and medications like it work, with minimal side effects. As Elizabeth Wurtzel says, depression "ruins…lives," [27] and deserves the same attention as cancer or heart disease. Jeanne Fahnestock would see the drug companies as "science accommodators" [126]. She notes that there are two basic appeals in an ethical argument, such as persuading someone that they may have depression. The appeals are "the wonder" and "the application" [126]. The wonder is that one may be depressed, and the application is the drug, such as Prozac, which will allow a return to everyday life. Critical of science accommodators, she says that "accommodators will leap to results, whereas the original authors stay on the safe side of the chasm" [126]. But this is precisely why DTC advertising is important.

DTC advertising breaks down the mystery of heavy scientific language and makes it understandable. "Comorbidity in disruptive mood regulation disorder" [100] does not ring with the average consumer. We need the drug companies to accommodate us and make the issue clear, thus a dumbing down of scientific language, which some see as manipulative. Many famous scientific writers, such as Michio Kaku, write for a general audience to make their complex research and findings discernible to the general public. Otherwise, we have valuable and very interesting information that remains out of reach. Few laypersons can fathom an article in a peer-reviewed physics journal, but can grasp a book by Kaku, which requires much effort and discipline to create for the average reader. A critique by Fahnestock is this ability to be clear and interesting: "The pressure to be interesting is only one explanation of the changes in statement types and purpose that occur between scientific report and scientific popularization" [126]. DTC advertising thus seeks to be interesting while conveying the basic facts, which is good for consumers.

A final criticism from Ryan is that DTC ads promote the idea that "Life has to be perfect, otherwise we are depressed. This definition of happiness is unattainable because it is unrealistic, and yet, the companies are trying to sell this definition—and succeeding" [32]. Treating depression does not guarantee a perfect life. Promising "a return to normalcy" does not insinuate a perfect life. The ads do promote an aspect of normalcy, which is problematic and hard to quantify, but ultimately, the idea is to make life more livable. Ryan adds, "While these advertisements seem to be giving the viewer control over becoming a patient-consumer, they are actually exploiting our desire to know our bodies" [32]. Wanting to know one's body is a great thing, though. Entering a doctor's office armed with knowledge about a particular disease benefits the doctor-patient relationship, which can often be heavily weighted toward the authority of the doctor. Knowledge is power and may make physicians leery, but consumers have the right to know about depression and its treatment, even if all they know is from a drug advertisement.

Much data has been published on the cost of DTC advertising, and the dollars being spent are large. It has been noted that drug companies must invest significantly in a drug to bring it to market. For a drug to be approved by the FDA, it must show an advantage over placebo in at least two double-blind, controlled studies, which cost millions of dollars. According to Charles Barber, "Of the eighty thousand clinical trials conducted in the

United States in a typical year, fifty thousand to sixty thousand are industry-sponsored" [22]. The adage that you have to spend money to make money holds true, and DTC advertising is not cheap.

Following the relaxing of rules by the FDA for DTC advertising in 1997 up to 2005, "spending on direct-to-consumer advertising tripled from $1.1 billion to $4.2 billion [127]. According to Meredith B. Rosenthal et al., "such advertising accounts for only 15 percent of the money spent on drug promotion and is highly concentrated on a subgroup of products" [124]. "Television ads accounted for the bulk—$1.1 billion—of the expenditure, up 70 percent from 1998" [122]. Relaxing the rules certainly played a role in this increase of spending, but we also have to consider that there was an increase in the number of effective medications being made available [124]. Regarding the advertising of the SSRI Paxil, a cousin of Prozac, "In 2000, GlaxoSmithKline spent $91.8 million...(more than Nike spent on advertising sneakers!) to make it the fourth most heavily promoted prescription drug in America" [32].

Despite the rise in DTC advertising, "promotion to health care professionals still accounts for more than 80 percent of the money spent on the promotion of prescription drugs" [124]. This seems to be a good sign from the drug companies, showing that they are not entirely focused on blitzkrieging the American consumer and are trying to ensure that physicians are familiar with the medications they prescribe. Another cost related to DTC advertising is screening for depression, which raises the hackles of many [106]. Elliott criticizes screening efforts as a false effort to appear like "grass-roots patient support" [39]. He describes National Depression Awareness Day as a media event pushed by big pharma:

Depression Since Prozac—Finding the True Self

National Depression Awareness Day began in 1991 and is now a national media event. In October of each year, hospitals and universities around the country offer free depression screening. People are encouraged to dial twenty-four-hour 800-numbers and take an automated depression screening test. At the end of the test, a computer analyzes the score and tells the person the severity of his or her symptoms. Who pays for the press kits, the 800-numbers, and the depression screening kits? Eli Lilly, the manufacturer of Prozac. [39]

But who else is going to pay for this? Does it matter who pays for it? The important thing is that those needing treatment receive it.

Ultimately, marketing antidepressants is a matter of business. How else will drug companies distribute their medications through the vast distribution chains of consumer products? Consumers deserve to know about the available options to treat a debilitating illness. Of course, therapy is an option and should be part of a physician's balanced approach to depression treatment, but therapy as a product is hard to define. One can't buy therapy at the local drug store. Perhaps ads for Prozac should mention therapy as an option or as an adjunct therapy, but from a marketing standpoint, the message becomes diluted and harder to digest. It is up to physicians to guide the patient toward the most appropriate treatments. What matters most is that people who are depressed have easy access to treatment, and DTC advertising and marketing to physicians, despite the reek of capitalism, is a vital part of that process.

Prozac and Creativity

Does Prozac make you more creative, or does it drain you of that life force? Many think that medications like Prozac take away personality, take one's true self, and that creativity will suffer as a consequence. Carl Wilson says that "people must suffer for beauty" [26]. But can't one still suffer while on Prozac? It is certainly not a cure, and one's basic personality does not change. One simply feels better. If anything, Prozac makes it more possible to create versus lying in bed all day thinking about how awful life is.

Anna Moore asks: What if Van Gogh had taken Prozac? "Perhaps he'd have given up art and become a life coach. Another possibility is that we'd now have more of his paintings" [17]. That more or less sums it up. One never knows what the other course would have been like, but as with many victims of depression, Van Gogh led a tumultuous life that came to a bad end. Many writers suffer from depression, perhaps at a higher rate than the general population. Peter Kramer says, "As for literature, studies indicate that an astonishing percentage, perhaps a vast majority, of serious writers are depressives" [45]. Kimberly Emmons expands on this, saying that depression "is an illness saturated with language; it inspires nearly compulsive storytelling" [56]. Charles Barber mentions Emily Dickinson as "the poet laureate of melancholy," referring to the first line from one of her poems: "'I felt a funeral in my brain'" [22]. Praising the value of sadness, he says that "[melancholia] becomes a muse of understanding, of insight into the secret kinship between antinomies" [26]. It certainly is the case that many with depression draw inspiration from their condition, but how much better might they work if treated?

Depression Since Prozac—Finding the True Self

Tennessee Williams famously said, "If I lose my demons, I will lose my angels as well." But, is this born out of a lack of experience with feeling well? Living with untreated mental illness is brutal, and one can't think beyond it. Wilson ponders Carl Jung, saying that "melancholia and insight are intimately connected, that profound gloom generates rapid light, that dissolution is the key to transformation" [26]. But, untreated depression will dissolve a person, perhaps to suicide. Quoting Virginia Woolf from a letter to Ethel Smith in 1930, Wilson shares this: "'As an experience, madness is terrific...and not to be sniffed at, and in its lava I still find most of the things I write about'" [26]. Woolf wrote brilliant novels, such as *Mrs. Dalloway,* and was indeed suffering from depression, drowning herself in the River Ouse in 1941. Had she been treated, what other great works would she have composed? We'll never know.

If we are speaking of serious depression, major depressive disorder, the disease is capable of driving one down into oblivion. Says Foucault, who lumps mental illness as madness, "In Shakespeare or Cervantes, madness still occupies an extreme place, in that it is beyond appeal. Nothing ever restores it to either truth or reason. It leads only to laceration and thence to death" [58]. One may write a great novel along the way, as did suicide victim John Kennedy Toole, who wrote *A Confederacy of Dunces,* or Sylvia Plath, who wrote *The Bell Jar.* Creative people are certainly capable of spinning the fantastic into reality, but when it is only illness that one operates under, that is a sad life.

So, there must be creativity whether on medication or not. Lots of creative people take Prozac and medications like it. Says Moore, speaking of depression, manic-depression, schizophrenia, obsessive-compulsive disorder, and anxiety disorders, "When patients are acutely ill, these psychiatric disorders block creativity" [34]. Truly sick, the most creative person is rendered helpless, and productivity declines or stops. Gwyneth Lewis recounts how depression affected her writing:

> After a severe episode of depression, which kept me home from work for most of a year, colleagues repeatedly asked me, 'We're you writing?' For a good deal of my sick leave, I'd been unable to lift my pen, get out of bed, or speak for more than a minute or two...So no, I wasn't writing, but I was making mental notes. [128]

And perhaps it is these mental notes that one makes while depressed that later turn into a work of genius. It is hard to say. But if one has the choice of being sick or not sick, regardless of the creative outcome, it seems that one would want to be well and draw on that strength for perhaps something different but still genius. Barbara Lefcowitz notes, "But overall, the integration of poetry and therapy has been, and continues to be, a definite plus in terms of clarifying feelings and ideas and, especially, expanding them, thus enhancing whatever talents I have" [129].

Prozac can lead you from dysfunction to something perhaps greater than could be imagined. Susan Squier says, "I do understand Prozac as compatible with a certain kind of spiritual journey" [103]. This is a journey that could not be taken without medication. Sick with depression, one is miserable and makes those nearby miserable as well. Ghaemi notes, "To many, the world is a flat and soulless place. It is a land in which to despair, a land for the already dead, pretending to be alive" [7]. This is the land of depression. If "culture sets limits of tolerance for specific emotions and strong affect..." [42], then culture should be as alarmed at the prostrate poet as at the painter suffering from a bout of mania. Creative types tend to press beyond society's limits and find refuge in their calling. But one doesn't have to be operating at extremes to draw or write well. Tod Chambers rightly asks, "Are we a nation that loves the sick soul and thus treasures the intellectual, aesthetic, or religious offspring of the spiritual struggle" [130]? At root, we probably are, and to the detriment of many talented people trying to make their way against depression. Discussing James Joyce's epiphany, Lionel Trilling says that "human existence is in largest part compounded of the dullness and triviality of its routine, devitalized or paralysed by habit and the weight of necessity..." [50]. Life indeed is hard at times, and depression compounds that hardness, often into something unendurable.

Missing one's demons and failing creatively seems unlikely, but if it were somehow true, there are tradeoffs. One has to see the bigger picture, like Ron Powell:

> I found, and find, inspiration for poetry at the edges of that emotional continuum [manic depression]. When I'm on medication I do sometimes miss the fuzzy hallucinations and emotional highs. And yet, without the clarity that medication has afforded me, I don't think I could write the poems. [131]

If you are functioning within that realm of despair, it doesn't mean that your work will reek of dismay. Of course, depression may manipulate the content of an artist's work. But, J.D. Smith says, "Being a poet in despair does not necessarily make one a poet of despair" [132]. And often it is the need to see beyond oneself that medication affords. Smith observes:

> The depression that had mercifully turned me away from gregarious and time-consuming professions such as selling real estate or running for office, which might have distracted me from poetry altogether, had also kept me from paying sufficient attention to subjects beyond myself and

focusing those lenses on topics other than myself is a growing source of pleasure for me. [132]

Withdrawn into the sick role, the world narrows, and attention to larger matters shrinks. Liza Porter reflects on the expansive effects of antidepressants: "After the antidepressants begin to work, my work becomes more universal. Others besides me can relate to it. I have energy to submit poems to magazines. Editors begin accepting them" [133]. The title of a poem by Smith is instructive: "Overshadowed by a blade of grass." So much is lost in the dark shade of depression. Powell adds, "There are those who hold that the true artist is not only allowed but obligated to indulge in excesses…for the sake of art" [131]. Some might say that this translates into a kind of mad focus, and that may be true, but at what cost? Taking medication, as I argue elsewhere, does not change the fundamental nature of the self or the soul. According to Lewis, "You can't manipulate a poet who's fully committed to writing because he or she is listening to a subtle but compelling rhythm that is linked to his or her most authentic self" [128]. Jack Coulehan finds that on medication, his true self is still accessible:

> The other surprising feature [in addition to productivity] was that I didn't experience myself as different—that is, my feelings were different, but the 'I' that had those feelings was the same Jack that had always been there, only richer in texture and more authentic. [134]

And the healthy self—the self on medication—is the true self. Medication can more sharply define the authentic self and enable a fuller, more robust life. Taking Prozac is, thus, not an act of deception, but an act of authenticity. Says Lionel Trilling, "The deception we best understand and most willingly give our attention to is that which a person works upon himself" [50]. In other words, it is the conscious act of duplicity that renders one inauthentic, not the restoration of sanity by medication.

Medication for depression and other mental illnesses lifts and restores energy. Writer Thomas Krampf, who lives with schizophrenia, observes: "If there was one difference characteristic of my writing and my creativity before and after psychiatric intervention, it was the ability to tap into some of these blind channels of energy and turn...to get out of them before I got hurt" [135].

Powell is hopeful, on medication, when he says, "No, I'm not saying that I write as well as Bukowski or Plath, but I'm not dead. I may yet write a masterpiece" [131]. Taking Prozac does not shut down the channels of creativity and offers one the fundamental right of living. Thomas Krampf says, "I am firmly convinced had I not found a reliable means of 'coping' with my disease, any further writing would have been out of the question" [135]. Productivity is a means of satisfaction for creative types, as well as for us all. And, depression decreases productivity.

We can't all be as productive as Honoré de Balzac, whose complete works span forty-eight volumes in one publisher's complete set, or Joyce Carol Oates, who has penned over one hundred novels. But Prozac and medications like it will increase one's ability to create. Time wasted brooding on death or fascinated with despair is dissipated. Says Renee Ashley, "I do not write during the bad times; I write on the upswing—but I have tried to capture what depression is, how it feels. It does not feel creative" [136]. Says Caterina Eppolito of her disorder,

> Anorexia is so consuming that one doesn't have the energy or strength to be creative or prolific. During the progression of the illness, I had begun a journal with the idea that I could capture on the page what I was mentally experiencing. But as the illness became more and more severe, my

writing diminished in the same way my body did. [137]

But society wants to hold the artist's feet to the fire of Foucault's madness. It often seems that we expect the writer, sculptor, or painter to be living at the edge of sanity, that that is a requirement. According to poet Edward Hirsch, "Implicit in poetry is the notion that we are deepened by heartbreak, that we are not so much diminished as enlarged by grief..." [138]. Powell, while working with a group of actors, notes, "It was obvious that, in their eyes, my mental disorder [manic depression] gave me clout as an artist" [131]. Vanessa Haley expounds on this expected role of artists to be "crazy": "Creativity occurs when I allow a dissolution of self and access the primitive psychic fears and longings hovering just beyond anxiety's sharp edges..." [138]. But accessing one's psychic fears does not go away with Prozac. They are still there, and the soul is perfectly able to access them in a productive way. David Budbill, who saw the value in his depression, says, "Clearly, or so it seemed to me, poetry and depression were lovers doing some kind of macabre dance in and with my life, and I was, it appeared, helpless..." [139]. When depressed, one has to fight and can often do great things, but ultimately, there is that feeling of helplessness that prevails, which limits the ability to create.

Giving up this helplessness, this well of despair from which one imagines his creativity emerges, is often not easy. The artist becomes used to operating in the sick role and holds onto it dearly. Says Elizabeth Wurtzel, "I had fallen in love with my depression...I loved it because I thought it was all I had" [27]. One can even feel guilty for seeking treatment and losing the bonds of depression. Jesse Millner brings up the idea that taking Prozac is a form of cheating society, which is a popular notion among writers such as Charles Barber, Joseph Glenmullen, and Carl Elliott.

Depression Since Prozac—Finding the True Self

Says Millner,

> I tell her [his therapist] I feel guilty for taking Prozac, which seems to be helping but feels like cheating" [140]. But he notes that he is free of his suicidal thoughts, although "the voice within that reminds me I'm a piece of shit still whispers in dark moments. [140]

What are the characteristics of a creative person? Albert Rothenberg has studied the creative state in *Creativity and Madness: New findings and Old Stereotypes.* He examines the qualities of creativity and discusses the role of mental illness in the creative process. Ultimately, he says that "Creativity is, therefore, the production of something that is both new and truly valuable" [141]. Regarding the personality traits of the creative types he observes, he says:

> Creators are neither generally compulsive nor impulsive, although many—even highly outstanding ones, interestingly—are somewhat rigid, meticulous, and perfectionistic rather than free or spontaneous. Some degree of introversion—inwardness and self-preoccupation—does predominate among creative people in many fields, but some are surprisingly extroverted. [141]

These seem to be quirks of the creative type that are geared toward productivity, but not the disabling features, such as suicidal thinking, that come with depression. To be creative, one has to bend the mold and see things simultaneously through a microscope and a telescope and bring together the confusion into a coherent whole.

Regarding mental illness and creativity, Rothenberg has found that "key aspects of creative thinking have nothing really to do with psychosis. They consist of healthy thought processes that generally arise from healthy minds" [141]. Thus, the artist wallowing in depression as necessary to create is a stereotype versus a reality. An artist should not put so much weight on her disease as to avoid treatment. Rothenberg states that "justifying avoidance of treatment on the basis that psychotic suffering is necessary for creativity is unwarranted" [141], which is good news for the depressed.

Rothenberg cools to that idea of the irrational and troubled soul as a repository of genius: "[T]he truly creative person is oriented toward producing something outside of himself, is rational, and is completely aware of logical distinctions" [141]. Under the weight of severe or even moderate depression, this ability to be rational is often absent. He further states that "they cannot be psychotic at the time they are engaged in a creative process, or it will not be successful" [141]. Rothenberg tells us, based on his decades of experience with creative types, that there is no specific "working pattern" that creatives have in common, but that the number one and only characteristic that makes a creative person successful is motivation [141]. He has formulated an idea called the janusian process and has this to say about works of genius that emerge from artists:

> The janusian process lies at the heart of the most striking creative breakthroughs...In the janusian process, multiple opposites or antitheses are conceived simultaneously, either as existing side by side or as equally operative, valid, or true. In an apparent defiance of logic of physical possibility, the creative person consciously formulates the simultaneous operation of antithetical elements or factors and develops those formulations into integrated entities and creations. [141]

Depression Since Prozac—Finding the True Self

We need motivation to succeed as artists and reach for genius. One thing lacking among the depressed is exactly that motivation. One can't get out of bed. It is a very simple and crippling factor of the illness, but so pervasive that it ultimately buries any motivation that may exist except during brief periods of lucidity. Participating in Rothenberg's janusian process requires clear faculties and the energy and state of mind to bring chaos into order and create something new, to create art.

Many writers write about depression and do so with lucid precision. One such writer is William Styron, who writes of depression as "a sense of self-hate...a general feeling of worthlessness...dank joylessness...a failure of self-esteem..." [21]. In Goethe's opening to *The Sorrows of Young Werther,* a letter to the reader, describes a similar condition that Young Werther finds himself in:

> Sorrow and discontent had taken deep root in Werther's soul, and gradually imparted their character to his whole being. The harmony of his mind became completely disturbed; a perpetual excitement and mental irritation, which weakened his natural powers, produced the saddest effects upon him, and rendered him at length the victim of an exhaustion against which he struggled with still more painful efforts than he had displayed, even in contending with his other misfortunes. [24]

Published in 1902, this is a prescient and worthy description of depression as captured by a great artist of that day.

Much popular writing also examines depression. The memoirs *Prozac Nation* and *Prozac Diary* became best-sellers. Sylvia Plath's *The Bell Jar* is a classic portrayal of depression. Much young adult fiction has of late concerned itself with self-harm and suicide, such as *Thirteen Reasons Why* and *The Perks of Being a Wallflower*. Literary journals burst at the seams with stories, essays, and poems of depression and mental illness. A short story in *Crazyhorse* called "Summers Off" by Jacob White is an excellent rendering of the depressed state of mind. Here is an excerpt reprinted with permission from the author:

> The need to get a hold on the day, finally: the imperative persists despite mind-flounder. The week of teaching has run through me like so many watery beers, leaving in me a tiredness filmed by inarticulate shame. It is Thursday, I've got nothing tomorrow, but I am afraid to get buzzed, or I am just not very interested, or too tired. My subconscious grew up, went impotent.
>
> In the kitchen, I open a beer left by some students a few weeks back, and it is terrible. Blue Moon? What adult drinks this perfume? But it ballasts me in a way I had not expected, and that is agreeable and warrants finishing, which increases the ballast even at the expense of brain blur, Aztec rug blur. I drift rudderless over the rug and accept the couch. I would be okay with some ice cream.
>
> To think now, there was a part of me that saw at the eye of all this impending horror of their departure some excitement of living alone, finally—as if then, at last, I might unspring with productive hobbies and indulgences, allowing my mind to crumble out the minutes with tinkering and reading and stuff. But I remain as dull to myself now as I'd been under her oppressive disappointment, and the loneliness only makes me see my reflection all the clearer. I am everything she said I was, only smaller.

Depression Since Prozac—Finding the True Self

There is no ice cream. I summon muster for a laundry errand to the basement. The transactions of washed and unwashed, the sorting—I can fathom none of it intellectually right now. I am trusting that I will know what to do when I get down there.

I am having to think too much. I have think exhaustion. My serotonin is having trouble covering the miles. It is tired of these daily forced pilgrimages. Take me out to the ball game. Take me out. [142]

That's a great line: "There is no ice cream," which sums up well the mundane weight of depression in an everyday setting. One feels as if there is no ice cream in life, that there is no flavor to life, and that life can seem unbearable in even the most minor details.

Depression, ultimately, is detrimental to the creative process, limiting productivity and motivation. Even on Prozac, there will still be remnants of the depression, and one may still plunge during a stressful time. Lessons learned from sadness are still available to anyone, regardless of medication status. Some artists, as did Wurtzel, may develop a kind of love affair with their depression, having learned to live with it, and feel that it is necessary for their art. Like a character in the novel *Martereau: A Novel*, "I felt all of a sudden that I had not really lived, I wanted to throw myself headlong into life, I wanted to struggle, really suffer..." [143]. There is value in struggle and bouts of sadness that enrich one's life, but the diseased form of this sadness that accompanies despair is beyond what is useful from life's ups and downs

But one still has hope during bouts of depression, whether treated or not. Budbill reflects, "I've come to understand my periods of depression not as useless periods in my life, periods that are to be fought against and resisted, but as dormancy periods, gestation periods, to be accepted, given in to, welcomed" [139]. This is great, as long as the depression does not overwhelm, which is most often the case with true depression and not idle sadness at bad weather. Again, there is that fear that Prozac will somehow interfere with creativity. Coulehan says, "My greatest fear, however, was that taking the drug [an SSRI] would diminish creativity. In retrospect, this fear was ridiculous; I had written very little poetry in the preceding six months..." [134]. So, we must not fear Prozac and medications like it. We must not fear that we will lose something vital to oneself. Treated and free of disease, the artist, like others, will experience the vitality to create and possibly produce that desired work of genius, that depression may diminish.

Poet T.S. Eliot said that "The progress of an artist is a continual self-sacrifice, a continual extinction of personality" [144]. The artist is concerned with expressing his creativity and leaving a lasting impact through his method. Art is that which requires a second and third look, perhaps a continuous look. Creating is a form of self-sacrifice, as Eliot notes, and involves the yielding of one's life forces to the creative project at hand. Suffering from depression, this arduous task may not be possible or yield incomplete results. James Joyce said that "The personality of the artist...finally refines itself out of existence..." [145]. This somewhat mysterious reference calls on the artist to put everything available into their works, to push beyond mediocrity and create lasting art. One needs every resource available, including sanity, to truly accomplish art.

Creativity may certainly dance with depression at times, but ultimately, the fatigue of depression limits the ability to enact creativity. Avoiding medications such as Prozac, hoping for the next masterpiece dragged through the mire of depression, is a hapless maneuver. But society places value on the suffering depressed artist even if that artist succumbs to the ultimate sacrifice of suicide. We need to place more value on the artist as a healthy, living being rather than a crippled muse serving some sadistic artistic need.

Suicide

In his autobiographical novel *The Turning Point,* Klaus Mann answers the question "Why does someone commit suicide?" and says this: "Because one will not, cannot go through the next half hour, the next five minutes. Suddenly, one comes to a dead end, the point of death. The limit has been reached..." [146].

The taking of one's life is a preventable disaster [10]. Consistently over the past few decades, suicide has ranked number ten overall in the United States as a leading cause of death. From 4 suicides per 100,000 in 1950, the United States suicide rate increased to 14 per 100,000 by 1990 [147], and the rate continues to increase despite the introduction of the SSRIs such as Prozac. The reasons for this are unknown, but there are hypotheses that increased suicides have resulted from a variety of factors, such as earlier onset of puberty in girls and the increasing inundation of life with information via social media, cell phones, gaming, and the Internet. It is also possible that an increased awareness of depression and suicide has helped to label questionable deaths as suicides, whereas earlier they may have been reported as accidents. Between 1980 and 2014, unintentional injuries increased 29 percent, ranking fourth as an overall cause of death [148]. However, in the same period, suicides nearly doubled, remaining the tenth leading cause of death [148]. It could be that increased awareness of depression and suicide moved unintentional injury cases to the category of suicide. And, perhaps this is obvious, had we not had medications such as Prozac, the suicide numbers could be even higher.

According to the Centers for Disease Control and Prevention (CDC), in the United States, "In 2013, suicide was the second leading cause of death among persons aged 15–24 years, the second among persons aged 25–34 years, the fourth among persons aged 35–54 years…" [8]. Overall, "the risk of dying from suicide was more than double for the white population than for the black population" [149]. Suicide is accomplished in various ways, but the primary method for males is by firearm. More firearm deaths occur annually as a result of suicide than homicide. According to the CDC, "The two major component causes of firearm injury deaths in 2013 were suicide (63.0 percent) and homicide (33.3 percent)" [149]. Nationally, suicide represents 2.2 percent of all deaths across all groups. Heart disease leads the causes at 31.7 percent [150].

In general, men are four times more likely to commit suicide than women, but "women are more likely to express suicidal thoughts and to make nonfatal attempts than men" [8]. And, "Suicide ranks as the number one cause of mortality in young girls between the ages 15 and 19 years globally" [151]. According to Diekstra, "In almost all countries the highest suicide rates are among elderly men (age category 75+)" [147].

Suicide is expensive. Reported by the CDC, "Suicides result in an estimated $44.6 billion in combined medical and work loss costs" [8]. The average suicide costs a staggering $1,164,499 [9]. Here are a few more facts about suicide in the U.S.

More than 40,000 people died by suicide in 2012.

More than 1 million people reported making a suicide attempt in the past year.

More than 2 million adults reported thinking about suicide in the past year.

Most people who engage in suicidal behavior never seek mental health services. [9]

Every forty seconds, someone in the world takes their life [10]. Globally, "an estimated 804,000 suicide deaths occurred worldwide in 2012, representing an annual global age-standardized suicide rate of 11.4 per 100,000 population (15.0 for males and 8.0 for females)" [10]. According to Diekstra, "In some countries, such as Denmark and Japan, suicide is even the number one cause of death in the age group 25-34" [147]. Diekstra also notes that "at least 10 times as many persons make a non-fatal suicide attempt or deliberately harm themselves" [147].

As in the United States, globally, "Social, psychological, cultural and other factors can interact to lead a person to suicidal behaviour, but the stigma attached to mental disorders and suicide means that many people feel unable to seek help" [10]. In the U.S, a variety of agencies work at suicide prevention, including the CDC and the National Institute of Mental Health (NIMH) in the public sector and groups such as the National Alliance on Mental Illness (NAMI) in the private sector. A goal of the WHO's "Mental Health Action Plan 2013–2020" is a reduction of 10 percent in the suicide rate. The "Plan" seeks to "provide support and appropriate referrals to those in need of assistance, families and social circles, enhance resilience, and intervene effectively to help loved ones" [10]. The "Plan" also seeks to foster "a social climate where help-seeking is no longer taboo and public dialogue is encouraged" [10]. Encouraging people to talk about their depression and suicidal thoughts and providing effective treatment is key to lowering the suicide rate worldwide. S.A. Montgomery et al. say, "Suicidal thoughts are a particularly worrying aspect of depression and any reduction, particularly early in treatment, is welcome" [14].

Antidepressants such as Prozac are key to treating suicidal

thoughts and actions, although the drug can increase suicidal thoughts, as warned by the FDA, especially among children and adolescents. In 2004, "the Food and Drug Administration required drug companies to amend antidepressant labels with a prominent warning of increased risk of suicidal thinking in children and adolescents" [152]. Some might point to Dan Blazer's statement as affirming that risk: "From 1970 to 1997, suicide rates among adolescents in the United States...tripled, even as rates of other age groups declined..." [57]. This would exclude the SSRIs as a possible cause before 1987. In 2006, "an advisory committee to the FDA recommended that the agency extend the warning to include young adults up to age 25" [15]. It is thought that this response of suicide to the SSRIs is due to the energizing effect of the antidepressant. Prior to treatment, one simply didn't have the energy to carry out a suicidal act. Also, it is usually the most depressed who are treated. Maurizio Fava and Jerrold F. Rosenbaum suggest that improvement enables a patient to become "mobilized to carry out suicidal ideation" [153]. A second explanation is the "rollback phenomenon" postulated by T.P. Dete and H.G. Jarecki in 1971: "As the depressive illness remits, it recapitulates in reverse order many of the stages and symptoms that were seen during the time it developed" [154]. Montgomery et al. (1995) note that

> antidepressants are prescribed on the assumption that they will improve the depression; suicidal thoughts, which are part of depression, should improve as the depression improves. Concerns are however expressed that antidepressants may paradoxically worsen certain symptoms, for example open anecdotal reports have described a development or worsening of suicidality or suicidal thoughts associated with fluoxetine [Prozac] therapy. [14]

This is a real risk, and newcomers to medications such as Prozac should alert their caregivers if such an adverse reaction occurs. However, the bottomless pit of depression, where one wallows in misery and thinks of death daily, begs for treatment, which Prozac and medications like it provide.

What is the link between suicide and serotonin? Montgomery et al. report that "Some post-mortem studies found lower levels of 5-hydroxyindoleacetic acid (5-HIAA), the primary metabolite of serotonin, in the brains of suicide victims compared with controls" [14]. According to M.T. Walsh and G.T. Dinan (2001),

> It has been recognized since the early 1970s that reduced levels of 5-HIAA [the metabolite of serotonin] in CSF [cerebrospinal fluid] often occurs in depression...It was recognized subsequently that in depressed patients with low 5-HIAA there were significantly more suicide attempters than in patients with normal 5-HIAA [79].

Thus, it seems there is a way to prevent suicides by raising the levels of brain serotonin, which is what the SSRIs such as Prozac and Paxil do: "Paroxetine [Paxil] showed an advantage in reducing suicidal thoughts in all analyses compared with placebo" [14]. Thus, taking an antidepressant is better than taking a placebo, although many argue that antidepressants work no better than placebo. In drug studies of depression treatments, it is often the case that suicidal individuals will be eliminated from the study, biasing the drug's efficacy if using suicide as an outcome [14].

From a United Kingdom study of 172,598 people in 1995 to "estimate the rate and means of suicide among people taking ten commonly prescribed antidepressant drugs," researchers found that 143 people committed suicide. "The overall rate of suicide was estimated to be 8.5 per 10,000 person years" [83]. Of those 143 who committed suicide, 50 died from medication or substance overdose. In 8 of those 50, death was caused "exclusively or primarily by the antidepressant that they were taking at the time; all were taking tricyclic antidepressants" [83]. This highlights the great risk of death from tricyclics taken in an overdose and shows that no deaths occurred from overdosing on an SSRI. However, it was demonstrated by Susan Jick et al. that fluoxetine [Prozac] had the highest adjusted relative risk of suicide at 3.8, but the result was not statistically significant ($p<0.5$) [83]. So, the risk of suicide was highest with an SSRI, but there were no deaths as a result. They also noted, "People with a history of feeling suicidal or who had been prescribed multiple antidepressants were more likely to commit suicide than those with no such history" [83]. It appears that patients with a history of depression, being moved to the SSRIs from the older tricyclics, are already more prone to commit suicide, and that the SSRIs just happen to be the new medication. It is interesting to note that several pharmaceutical companies funded the study, except Eli Lilly and Company, the maker of Prozac.

In another well-known study by Charles Beasley et al., undertaken by scientists working for and funded by Eli Lilly, results of a meta-analysis of double-blind trials involving 3,065 patients showed that "data from these trials do not show that fluoxetine [Prozac] is associated with an increased risk of suicidal acts or emergence of substantial suicidal thoughts among depressed patients" [155]. Also, "Suicidal acts did not differ significantly in comparisons of fluoxetine with placebo (0.2 percent versus 0.2 percent, $p=0.494$)" [155]. Thus, at the time, it appeared that results were mixed depending on who was doing the research, with one group saying that Prozac increased suicidal behavior while another group said the opposite. In the Beasley et al. study, "those with a serious suicidal risk as clinically assessed by the investigator" were excluded from the study, as with the Jick et al.

study [155]. The prescription of SSRIs may reduce the toxicity of an antidepressant overdose, but it will not necessarily guarantee a lower suicide-attempt rate and, at worst, may cause the rate of suicide attempts to increase [156].

Another study from 2000 showed "Significantly more DSH [deliberate self-harm] events occurred following the prescription of an SSRI than that of a TCA (p<0.001). The occurrence of DSH was highest with fluoxetine [Prozac] and lowest with amitriptyline [Elavil]" [118]. The data resulted from 2,776 DSH cases, which did not, by definition, exclude persons with suicidal risk. Therefore, we have a much more potent subject population in which the focus is sharpened, limited to those who have already exhibited DSH.

In an effort to better understand the role of SSRIs in suicidal behavior, Stuart Donovan et al. uncovered some interesting insights. They examined 2,776 DSH cases presenting to emergency rooms, noting the medications patients were taking. Patients taking fluoxetine (Prozac) had the highest relative risk of 6.6 versus those taking amitriptyline; they were 6.6 times more likely to engage in DSH [118]. Furthermore, "Significantly more DSH events occurred following the prescription of an SSRI than that of a TCA (p<0.001)" [118]. But this must be balanced with the following:

> Equally relevant, however, is the pragmatic consideration that prescribers are heeding advice to prescribe safer-in-overdose antidepressants to patients who are perceived to be at greater risk of DSH. This effectively 'loads the dice' against antidepressants such as the SSRIs... [118]

And then again, "Furthermore, comprehensive analyses of clinical trial data do not support an association of increased suicide risk with fluoxetine" [79]. So, who to believe? Again, it is a choice of obtaining the best results for treating one's depression, but knowing that there are risks.

Reviewing data from 222 suicides who had been prescribed an antidepressant within the last month in the UK and Ireland, researchers found that only 32.9 percent were known to have depression in the past [156]. Thus, it is not a rule that one must be depressed to commit suicide, but we can infer that many of the 222 without a diagnosis of depression were, in fact, depressed. Also, being diagnosed and on treatment for depression does not guarantee that DSH will or will not occur, but the numbers could very well be much higher had no one in the study population been diagnosed or treated.

Donovan et al. also found that "suicide by any method...was more likely to occur following the prescription of SSRIs than of TCAs" [156]. This again is balanced by the finding that "less-overdose-toxic antidepressants were preferentially prescribed to patients at a higher risk of suicide..." [156]. This makes SSRIs more visible as methods of DSH than other medications. In effect, "The most likely explanation for the difference in suicidality between different antidepressants probably lies in selective prescribing" [156]. Kramer agrees, saying, "Prozac was safer in the hands of potentially suicidal patients who might attempt to overdose on the drug" [23]. Those who are sicker and more likely to commit suicide get the safer SSRIs versus the TCAs or MAO-Is, giving the impression that the SSRIs are more prone to lead to DSH. One cannot very well predict that a suicide will occur based on what treatment a person is receiving, but "numerous studies have shown that parasuicide [failing at suicide] is one of the most, if not the most powerful predictor of suicide" [147].

According to David Healy, based on clinical trials, "the SSRIs [are] no more effective in outpatient depression than were the older agents" [36]. Healy points to an older drug, phenelzine (an

MAOI), and notes that Sylvia Plath committed suicide one week after beginning the drug. Did she need more than a week's exposure? Was it too late in her depression for improvement? Would she have attempted suicide on an SSRI? If she had, she most likely would have survived. It is the older tricyclics and MAOIs that kill. Was her suicide solely reliant on the drug? Probably not. Plenty of people on antidepressants commit suicide, but even more would if antidepressants were not available and properly prescribed and taken for more than a week. Even Marilyn Tobias, the wife of a chief executive at Eli Lilly, the makers of Prozac, committed suicide after she began taking the drug [36].

Healy raises an interesting point when he notes that "mild depression might even confer some protection against suicide" [36]. But without treatment, mild depression may progress to severe depression, which is a kind of DSH. Healy suggests that the act of treating mild depression increases rates of suicide, but that is hard to prove. Healy calculated that the prescribing of Prozac led to 20,000 more suicides "over and above the number who would have committed suicide if they had been left untreated or been treated with older agents" [36]. That seems bold, knowing that most people who commit suicide are not on antidepressant medication. However, although clinical trials "offer no evidence for an increase in suicidal thoughts or suicide attempts from antidepressant treatment, it has been suggested that antidepressants may contribute to the risk of suicide in certain patients" [153]. Thus, medications such as Prozac can contribute to the risk of suicide, but do not in and of themselves cause suicide. For the vast majority who take the medications, the benefit of leading a happier and more productive life is the outcome and not suicide.

Further, in discussing data obtained from interviewing fellow clinicians, Fava and Rosenbaum (1991) found that "new-onset suicidal ideation" did not occur with fluoxetine [Prozac] and characterize that scenario as a popular ideation "of the intensity and severity described by Teicher and associates" [153]. In 1990, M.H. Teicher et al. published an alarming and now famous article ("The Teicher Report") in *The American Journal of Psychiatry*, reporting graphic case studies of persons who had become suicidal and violent after taking Prozac [116].

For example, a 62-year-old woman with a 17-year history of depression, having been treated with a variety of antidepressants, was prescribed fluoxetine [Prozac]. According to Teicher et al. "On day 11 [of treatment with Prozac] she began to experience forced obsessional suicidal thoughts consisting of intense and incessant wishes to kill herself" [116]. The patient felt that "death would be a welcome result" [116]. Another case involved a 39-year-old man with a 21-year history of dysthymia, but without a history of suicidal ideation. Thirty days after being prescribed fluoxetine (20 mg daily), the man was still severely depressed but "Most alarming, however, was the emergence of nearly constant suicidal preoccupation, violent self-destructive fantasies, and resignation...to the inevitability of suicide" [116]. Teicher et al. go on to describe four other cases with similar atypical responses to treatment with fluoxetine. The question arises, "Is the suicidal ideation a result of the fluoxetine not working or is it a result of the fluoxetine itself?" They end their paper by noting that "The purpose of this report is to suggest the surprising possibility that fluoxetine may induce suicidal ideation in some patients" [116]. That possibility is, of course, well documented, and there are now black-box warnings cautioning those taking medications such as Prozac.

One unanswered question is whether or not suicidal ideation would be even higher if no fluoxetine were prescribed or if perhaps the dose was not therapeutic. Fava and Rosenbaum note that inadequate doses of antidepressants could be a more pressing concern than the risk of suicidal ideation following said treatment [153].

Finally, we should all be worried about how to treat depression and prevent suicide. We have to throw the kitchen sink at it if required. A study by A.T. Beck et al. sought diagnostic criteria that would predict suicide among a sample of 207 patients who had been hospitalized due to suicidal ideation [157]. The team followed the cohort for 5 to 10 years and determined that 14 patients committed suicide. Diagnostic instruments given to all patients were then analyzed. The instruments included the Beck Depression Inventory (BDI) and a Hopelessness Scale. The study found that familial suicide and severity of depression did not predict suicide, but that the Hopelessness Scale and BDI did in a significant manner ($p<0.5$). According to Beck et al., "During the last 25 years hopelessness has emerged as an important psychological construct for understanding suicide" [157]. As an intervention, Beck et al. recommend therapies that reduce hopelessness to "lower suicidal potential" [157], including use of the SSRIs such as Prozac.

Suicide is a very real outcome, although minimal, of depression, and not being treated can result in acts of DSH. There is evidence that those taking SSRIs such as Prozac are more likely to engage in DSH, but often it is the case that they were put on the medications because of their existing risk. This stacks the odds against Prozac and medications like it. Suicide is devastating, but so are daily thoughts of suicide, which drain the soul of life. The SSRIs help provide relief from depressive symptoms and are an invaluable tool to maintain one's mental health. For those with nagging suicidal thoughts, sometimes described as racing thoughts of death, other medications such as an antipsychotic may prove very useful. Thus, Prozac is not a cure for depression or a guarantee against suicide, but is part of an effective regimen to minimize thoughts and acts of DSH, including suicide.

Therapy versus Antidepressants

Medications are but one arm of the body required to fight depression, although medications do work with or without therapy, the most common form being cognitive behavioral therapy (CBT). Of course, some patients do just fine with therapy alone, but for those with serious brain chemical imbalances, as with low serotonin or norepinephrine levels, medications work wonders. There is that worry, though, that taking an antidepressant reduces or obliviates the need for adjunctive psychosocial support [156]. We worry that a vital tool that touches on society is not being used. There is also that remnant of psychoanalysis remaining in this age of biological psychiatry that calls upon the self to adjust itself through confession. Many people want to talk about their illness and may be deprived of that with a single prescription.

The most practical approach to treating depression seems to be a combination of therapy and medication. Studying various combinations of treatment, I. Elkin et al. found "imipramine plus clinical management generally doing best, placebo plus clinical management worst..." [158]. There was no "evidence that either of the psychotherapies was significantly less effective than the standard reference treatment, imipramine plus clinical management" [158]. This study used an older antidepressant but indicates that drug therapy with clinical management reaps the best results, with psychotherapy alone coming in second and placebo doing the worst. Statistically significant differences among treatments were only present "for the subgroup of patients who were more severely depressed and functionally impaired" [158]. Thus, the sicker benefited the most from psychotherapy, but imipramine plus clinical management still prevailed overall. Clinical management differs from therapy and refers to office visits used to assess the effectiveness of the medications, usually every three months or more frequently if there is a medication change or worsening of depression.

In a study of the effectiveness of CBT, Jacqueline Persons et al. found that numerous randomized clinical trials of behavioral therapy for depression showed that it was more effective than no treatment and as effective as an antidepressant [159]. This does not hold true, though, for more serious depression, which responds best to pharmacotherapy. One key factor in whether CBT is prescribed is cost. Says Hacking, "Drugs, no matter how expensive, are much cheaper than long-term psychotherapy" [49].

Cognitive Behavioral Therapy

Persons et al. have written a seminal text on CBT and depression, and what follows relies heavily on their work. As the most common type of formal therapy for depression today, CBT is based on a variety of theories and in some way resembles psychoanalysis. However, CBT is less time-consuming and less expensive. The ideas of Aaron Beck, the recognized father of cognitive therapy, underlie Person et al.'s observations. I also make use of Mark Goldman's book, *Expectancy Operation: Cognitive-Neural Models and Architectures.*

Basically, Beck proposes that "depressive symptoms result when a vulnerable individual's maladaptive schema are activated by external life events...Schema are deep cognitive structures that enable an individual to interpret his or her experiences in a meaningful way" [159]. An example would be someone who thinks, "I am a bad person." Then, he hears that a friend has accused him of being devious. The result? Depression. The person has developed a schema: "I am a bad person," which is enforced by a life experience. Schemas, when activated, "produce negative mood, maladaptive behavior, and distorted thinking" [159]. These reactions to schema produce or contribute to the symptoms of depression. Thus, the patient in therapy will explore these schemas and adapt behaviors to counter them. An example would be expecting to become depressed around a major holiday because of hurtful past experiences. To counter this schema, the patient would develop a new way of viewing the holiday or even practicing the holiday to result in a more positive experience.

Therapy focuses on the behavior versus the mood itself because it "is easier to design interventions that target behaviors and cognition than to design interventions to target mood directly" [159]. This is juxtaposed with medications, which address the mood itself. One criticism of only treating with drugs is that these schema are not addressed and resolved, which makes patients "vulnerable to depression should the schema become activated at a later time" [159].

An important aspect of CBT is the concept of automatic behavior. Goldman notes that we view the world with "preexisting expectations about how the world is organized. It suggests that behavior influenced by these expectancies is most often not thought out in some deliberative fashion but is automatic in nature..." [160]. In more clinical language, "The term expectancy refers to dynamic information templates stored in the nervous system that are processed to produce behavioral output" [160]. Thus, the brain has been trained to respond in certain ways to stressors, and CBT seeks to retrain these responses and alter the templates. Through interventions aimed at these automatic thoughts, the "overt behavioral symptoms of depression can contribute to schema change" [159]. Patients are often encouraged to keep a thought journal where they record responses to these automatic thoughts. One becomes able to anticipate automatic reactions, known as response expectancies. An example would be someone who drinks a cup of coffee and expects to feel more alert. With depression, therapy guides the patient's response expectancies to anticipate a depressive response and seek to change that response, a kind of conditioning.

Less focused on the disorder itself, therapy does not necessarily follow a formulaic response based on the *Diagnostic and Statistical Manual of Mental Disorders (DSM)*. According to Persons et al., "Psychiatric diagnosis is not, strictly speaking, a component of a case formulation" [159]. Instead of being guided by symptoms of depression listed in the *DSM,* "A comprehensive problem list describes any problems the patient is having in any of the following domains: psychological-psychiatric symptoms, interpersonal, occupational, medical, financial, housing, legal, and leisure" [159]. Thus, the approach is more psychosocial than biological. Working together, the patient and therapist agree on treatment goals. The therapist is there to predict potential impediments and help the patient attempt to prevent or overcome them. One problem of this approach is that an unanticipated problem or predicament arises and "suddenly becomes a crisis" [159]. But the therapist seeks to be comprehensive in anticipating dilemmas, although it is time-consuming. According to Goldman, people seek understanding of their world and encode "aspects of their world, including aspects of themselves and other people. Such encoding, once formed, resists change and greatly influences the construal of subsequent events" [160], which the therapist must address deeply and thoughtfully.

Persons et al. note this tendency to take a slow and careful approach, using empathy as well as the therapist's problem-solving strategies [159]. This studied approach takes time and many meetings between patient and therapist. CBT distinguishes itself from other therapies through the use of "a carefully, explicitly structured therapy session" [159]. One aspect of this carefulness involves making the patient an active participant in the process through much homework, which results in better outcomes [159].

One example of such homework is activity scheduling. This gives structure to the patient's life and helps anticipate crises ahead. Interestingly, Persons et al. note that "some depressed patients experience little satisfaction because they spend most of their time doing things they do not enjoy" [159]. So, one goal is to schedule things they enjoy and work around things they do not enjoy, if possible.

CBT seeks to discover the why of depression—why patients "feel and behave the way they do" [159]. The therapist, with the big picture in mind, recognizes small steps and rewards each as an accomplishment. As depressed patients "are adept at punishing themselves," it is important for the empathetic therapist to be encouraging, practical, and to recognize the limits of a given patient [159]. Goldman observes that a patient's "cognitive abilities provide them with the tools for self-regulation. The capacity to envision goals allows people to create incentives that motivate and guide behavior" [160]. Says Persons et al., "Several studies show that patients treated with cognitive therapy are less likely to relapse than are patients treated with acute pharmacotherapy" [159].

Therapists working with CBT must become the eyes and ears of the patient, showing them their cognitive processes and resulting behaviors. Patients are often unaware of the ingrained templates in their brains that produce negative automatic behavior and ultimately depression. By working with new expectations to identify stimuli and stressors, a new, more productive behavioral response can be elicited. This takes much work, though, for the therapist and the patient. Says Goldman, "It is difficult for long-standing information patterns, which are continually strengthened by inherited physiological predispositions, to be easily changed" [160].

For those with the time and resources to explore CBT or another form of psychotherapy, the long-term benefits could be more pronounced than medication alone, although therapy plus medication seems best. At least, CBT positively reinforces healthy behavior and should make the medications more efficacious. However, for those not able or not inclined to therapy, medication alone for depression has been shown to work just as well [158]. Kramer says, "the effects of psychotherapy and antidepressant medications are not additive. For symptom relief, most of what medication and talk accomplish together can be done by medication alone" [23]. Although Shorter says, "This combination of psychotherapy plus medication represents the most effective of all approaches in dealing with disorders of the brain and mind" [18]. Given their resources and time, patients must decide which approach is best.

Psychoanalysis

Both psychotherapy, such as CBT, and psychoanalysis seek to change a patient's behavioral responses to stress and stimuli. The primary difference is that psychoanalysis focuses on the unconscious mind and its resistance to change, whereas psychotherapy seeks to alter behavioral templates in the brain. During its heyday, the 1940s, 50s, and 60s, psychoanalysis dominated the field of psychiatry, led by Sigmund Freud and his contemporaries and successors, but fell out of favor as biological psychiatry and psychiatry's desire to be more research-based gained traction. According to Foucault, Freud was the touchstone of all that followed from the nineteenth century's multiple paths to mental illness, then commonly referred to as madness. Foucault observes that it was Freud who was "the first man to accept in all its seriousness the reality of the physician-patient couple" and that he "demystified...asylum structures..." [58].

Although psychiatry was following a biological model set down by Emil Kraepelin in the 1890s,

> Freudian analysis shifted the center of gravity for psychiatric practice. Psychoanalysts treated patients with neuroses rather than psychoses—the worried well rather than inmates of the asylum. Increasingly, they saw middle-class patients in private clinics. [39]

According to van Praag, "Until well into the fifties long-term, individual, dynamic psychotherapy was the treatment modality in psychiatry, and psychoanalysis was the absolute gold standard of psychotherapy" [59]. Psychoanalysis sought to integrate the individual into the social system, whereas medication sought to restore proper biological function. Biological psychiatry, bolstered by medications that treated mental illness such as Thorazine and imipramine, called for more science than psychoanalysis could give, and psychoanalysis and Freud's "mysterious" unconscious waned [57]. Nasir Ghaemi says, "Much of our confusion about mental health...stems from continued Freudian influence" [7]. Certainly, psychoanalysis has given way to "real" psychiatry, but its influences and practice are still felt today.

Critical of psychiatry's path, Dan Blazer notes that where we once sought to find meaning and purpose, now we seek to find cures, largely through medications such as Prozac [57]. Eric Norden agrees, saying, "I have come to suspect that primary care doctors, perhaps from fear of offending their patients, actually avoid inquiring into their state of mind" (Norden, 1995). Ghaemi adds: "[A] search for psychoanalytic wisdom regarding mental health basically leads to an offhanded remark by Freud, who once defined the goal of successful psychoanalytic treatment to

Depression Since Prozac—Finding the True Self

be Arbeiten and Lieben: to work and to love" [7]. If you can't work or love, then you should do therapy. Regarding this shift from the social model of psychoanalysis to a biological model, Kramer notes,

> Perhaps medication now risks playing a role that psychotherapy was accused of playing in the past: it allows a person to achieve happiness through conformity to contemporary norms. This accusation is the 'mother's-little-helper' label in modern colors. [23]

With the new wave of biological psychiatry, clinical trial evidence became a mainstay. One could prove clinically that a drug worked in a specific manner, but this same rigor had never been applied to psychoanalysis. In the 1970s, demand for psychoanalysis declined. One reason for the decline was fueled by health maintenance organizations that balked at expensive long-term therapy. According to Shorter, by the 1990s, the "P" word, as he calls it, changed from psychoanalysis to Prozac [18].

So, there is excellent value in psychotherapy, specifically CBT, and patients suffering from depression need to have that treatment as an option. Some think that CBT alone is as effective as Prozac, but other research has shown that medications work just as well. Of course, psychotherapy is more expensive than medication, which can cost as little as five dollars a month. Healthcare providers would certainly love to have the business of psychotherapy, but healthcare insurance plans would rather not foot the bill, favoring cheaper medications with concomitant maintenance visits. With the second rise of biological psychiatry beginning in the 1950s and the discovery of psychiatric medications that worked, psychoanalysis began its slow decline in favor of research-based psychotherapy. There are still bastions of psychoanalysis, such as Argentina, which boasts the most psychologists per capita in the world, but treatment with medications such as Prozac, with or without psychotherapy, is king for now.

Depression Since Prozac—Final Words

The daily struggle against depression is relentless. Whether diagnosed or not, those suffering from depression suffer immeasurably, and relief is warranted. The most devastating outcome of depression is suicide, which in the United States is the second leading cause of death in those aged 15-34. Globally, depression is the number one cause of disability. As with cancer and heart disease, every effort to search for a cure and relief is deserved, and perhaps no better solution has arisen in the past 30 years than Prozac and medications like it.

Many minimize the importance of pharmacotherapy, thinking that taking medications such as Prozac renders a fatal blow to oneself, that taking medications is disingenuous, and that one's authenticity as a human being is undermined. However, authenticity is a state that is not reached through suffering but rather through finding peace and meaning in life, which depression robs.

Prozac, like no other drug before it, has brought much acclaim and disclaim, but ultimately has rendered depression a valid and real disease. Books such as *Prozac Nation* and *Prozac Diary*, mass media coverage in magazines and newspapers, and extensive scientific research have made depression an understandable, significant, and treatable disorder. There is no cure for depression, but medications such as Prozac work wonders and restore lives. We may worry that those on antidepressants become "better than well," but why wish others suffering? Prozac does not create superhumans with unfair superpowers but merely lifts one from a bog of confusion, whereby life can be lived as productively as those without depression. With the disease of depression present, the true self is the medicated self.

Depression "ruins...lives" [27]. It is estimated that 6.7 percent of Americans suffer from severe depression. Worldwide, 300 million suffer. Fifteen percent of Americans consider themselves not very happy, a rough indicator of depression, and half of the population with depression do not receive treatment. Depression causes severe psychological distress and may result in deliberate self-harm (DSH) and, at its worst, suicide. Suicide alone costs society an estimated $44.6 billion a year in combined medical and work loss costs.

The history of depression goes back to antiquity with the humors of Galen, which vaguely described the imbalance of melanchole or black bile as causing depression-like illness. Through the ages, melancholia became the general term for what we recognize as depression, and when persistent, it was often attributed to demonic possession. Lumped together with the general condition of madness, persons with melancholia often found themselves prisoners of asylums, where suffering was thought to be beneficial. In the nineteenth century, the idea that melancholia and other mental illnesses might be biological in nature came into being through the discovery of medications that worked against the symptoms of mental illness, such as the use of chloral hydrate as a hypnotic.

The diagnosis of mental illness as a disease process was spurred by the discovery of microorganisms that caused specific diseases, such as cholera, and specifically by the careful research and observations of Emil Kraepelin in the late 1890s, paving the way for the differential diagnosis of depression and other diseases based on empirical research. However, this biological psychiatry was soon overwhelmed by Freud and psychoanalysis, which

Depression Since Prozac—Finding the True Self

turned from a biological model of illness toward a model that placed disease in the mind. Depression was a neurosis to be battled through exploring sexual conflicts in the subconscious. With the discovery of new medications in the 1950s, such as Thorazine and the first antidepressants, there began a turning of the tide against psychoanalysis toward a renewed interest in biological psychiatry and a delineating of depression as a specific illness that responded well to medications that boosted neurotransmitter levels in the brain. This new focus on categories of mental illness as biological entities coincided with the rise of antipsychiatry in the 1960s, which claimed that this was just a clever way to trap patients into a diagnosis and bill insurance companies for dilemmas that were social versus medical.

Beginning in the 1970s, researchers isolated low brain serotonin as an important contributor to depression. After sixteen years in development, Prozac was released as a treatment for depression, and office visits for depression and prescriptions for depression soared. Critics of the SSRIs claimed this was disease mongering and that psychiatrists were on the hunt for depression now that an effective treatment was available. Prozac was even cited as making those treated "better than well," and the cry against it made it seem that Prozac somehow was unfair, akin to a nose job. Paralleling and guiding the rise of depression as a discrete illness, with variations, was the evolution of the *Diagnostic and Statistical Manual of Mental Disorders (DSM)*, which progressed from a handbook of disorders under the influence of psychoanalysis to a "Bible" of mental illnesses based on empirical research, with its latest edition, the fifth, published in 2013.

In the 1920s, the first neurotransmitter, acetylcholine, was discovered. In 1952, serotonin was discovered to be a neurotransmitter and soon linked to depression with the formation of the monoamine hypothesis that proposed "that patients with depression have depleted concentrations of serotonin, norepinephrine, and dopamine" [77]. Thus, research in the 1960s began to focus on finding medications that would increase the amount of these neurotransmitters available in the brain, leading to the first SSRI in 1972, zimelidine, which proved toxic, and then Prozac in 1987, which proved safe, efficacious, and easy to prescribe not only by psychiatrists but also by general practitioners. Side effects of these SSRIs have been noted, the most serious perhaps being sexual dysfunction. But as with any medication, one must weigh the benefits against the untoward side effects.

Prozac was an immediate success, grabbing headlines, some good and some bad. On the positive side, Prozac relieved symptoms of depression, such as sadness and feelings of unworth, and was safe in an overdose. A black-box warning was added in 2004 to the drug inserts of the SSRIs and other antidepressants that elevated neurotransmitter levels, warning of an increased risk of suicide in children, teens, and later in young adults. Following this warning, prescriptions for these medications dropped, leaving many untreated and vulnerable. But still, Prozac and medicines like it worked, and research indicated that they were safe.

One benefit of Prozac, specifically the generic forms of SSRIs, is its low price, available today for only $5 for a thirty-day supply. With clear criteria to diagnose depression provided by the *DSM* and cheap and effective medications that work, physicians were perfectly poised to meet a debilitating disease head-on. Prozac became a true celebrity and remains one of the most effective therapies for depression, often combined with psychotherapy for optimal results, although studies have shown that Prozac is as effective as therapy plus medication.

Prozac, of course, came under fire from many directions, with the results of clinical trials claiming that Prozac was no more effective than a placebo. The placebo effect has come under scrutiny by many, including Peter Kramer. A primary question is why a placebo would work better than Prozac. This can be explained in various ways. First, those on placebo may think they have received the real thing, which can make the placebo look equal to or better than the treatment. Second, those with mild depression who receive the treatment are already very close to "normal," making their progress minimal even though they may feel significantly better, giving placebo equal footing. Third, patients in a clinical trial may be non-responders to the medication, which makes the placebo look relatively good. Fourth, those receiving placebo also receive care and attention from the trial's raters. Often, persons participating in demanding clinical trials are poor and receive benefits such as payment, bus rides, and a comfortable environment in which to participate in the trial, which necessarily makes them feel better, even though on placebo. But, in the end, "Placebos don't prevent depression, and antidepressants do" [23].

The use of antidepressants for children and teenagers has drawn scrutiny, as it should. Parallels are drawn with children on Prozac and those being treated for ADHD. Prozac was approved for teens by the FDA in 2003, following 22 years of research and development, showing extreme caution. According to Mental Health America (2018), we have to remember that 8.2 percent of youth (or 1.9 million youth) have experienced severe depression at some point in their life [102]. And that does not mean just sadness but severe depression with symptoms of lethargy, self-loathing, despair, and possibly thoughts or acts of deliberate self-harm. Why should a child or teen have to wait to adulthood to be rid of a treatable disease? There is the concern, again, about an increase in suicidal thoughts once on an antidepressant, and the warnings of such a chance are made very clear, but that stands against the fact that the SSRIs in particular are very effective, ultimately bringing lasting relief regardless of age.

One reason for Prozac's success has been its marketing, specifically direct-to-consumer (DTC) advertising, although, in general, 80 percent of marketing costs are aimed at prescribers. There is much to criticize about big pharma foisting its wares on the public, but how else is the relief of depression with a simple medication to be broadcast? Should it simply be word of mouth? People need to know what depression is and how to treat it. One criticism of DTC advertising is that it objectifies the depressed as abnormal and that Prozac will restore one to "normal." However, to think of death daily is anything but normal, and bringing those thoughts to an end seems like a miracle, normal or not. Another criticism of drug marketing is that it creates the disease for which drug companies have the solution. However, depression has always existed, and marketing the disease only brings awareness, which is a good thing. It may be that a few who are genuinely not depressed find themselves on medication, but then there are the millions who truly have the disease and benefit from the medication. Despite the media coverage and marketing, millions remain untreated, and efforts to reach them should be continued.

Many worry that Prozac and medications like it will curtail creativity, especially among those whose profession hinges on some aspect of creativity, such as writers. This parallels the argument that medication robs one of the true self. The truth is that depression is the one doing the robbing. Under the influence of depression, one does not have the energy or fortitude to create and complete projects. If anything, antidepressants provide energy and insight, abetting the creative process. One's basic self is enhanced, and one's life is improved with treatment.

The specter of suicide looms as the ultimate sacrifice one pays to depression. Suicide rates have actually increased since the release of Prozac, but one can't fault the medication. Prozac and the SSRIs are very safe in overdose scenarios, but of course, firearms are not. More firearm deaths occur as a result of suicide than homicide, 63 percent to 3 percent. Numerous hypotheses exist as to why the suicide rate has increased, including an increased awareness of suicide and depression. Consistently over the past few decades, suicide has ranked number ten overall in the United States as a leading cause of death. The taking of one's life is cataclysmic and is preventable. The focus needs to remain on the causes of suicide, including depression and other mental illnesses, and the reduction of suicide.

Prozac or another antidepressant may be combined with psychotherapy, such as cognitive behavioral therapy (CBT), and with good results, although the medication alone has been proven to be as effective as medication plus therapy. Therapy is expensive and time-consuming, but many benefit from it and learn how to manage their depression by anticipating crises and learning how to react therapeutically. Psychoanalysis is still an option today, but it is costly and even more time-consuming than CBT. In the throes of a suicidal episode, one needs rapid treatment, as with medication, and therapy can follow.

Defining and treating depression today owes its efficiency to many factors, including the rise of biological psychiatry and the honing of diagnostic criteria through the *DSM*. But, perhaps, what has mattered most is the discovery of the SSRIs such as Prozac, which have provided a safe and easily prescribed medication for those suffering from depression. The public attention Prozac and depression have received is unprecedented and has resulted in depression and Prozac becoming a part of the vernacular. No longer is depression a fuzzy reaction or a madness instilled by demons, but it is a recognizable and treatable disease that the world has learned to embrace.

References

1. WHO Depression. Fact Sheet, 2017.
2. Pew Are we happy yet? 2006.
3. CDC Depression. 2017.
4. NIMH Major depression among adults. 2017.
5. Helliwell, J., R. Layard, and J. Sachs World happiness report 2017. 2017.
6. de Waal, A., Evil days: Thirty years of war and famine in Ethiopia. 1991, New York: Africa Watch.
7. Ghaemi, N., On depression. 2013, Baltimore: Johns Hopkins.
8. CDC Understanding suicide: Fact sheet. 2015.
9. CDC Suicide and suicide attempts take an enormous toll on society. 2016.
10. WHO, Preventing suicide. 2014, Geneva: World Health Organization.
11. WHO Suicide rates (per 100,000), by gender, USA, 1950-2005. 2005.
12. CDC Increase in suicide in the United States, 1999–2014. NCHS Data Brief, 2016.
13. NIMH Suicide. 2015.
14. Montgomery, S.A., D.L. Dunner, and G.C. Dunbar, Reduction of suicidal thoughts with paroxetine in comparison with reference antidepressants and placebo. European Neuropsychopharmacology, 1995. 5(1): p. 5-13.
15. NIMH Antidepressant medications for children and adolescents: Information for parents and caregivers. n.d.
16. NBC 'Black box' warning on antidepressants raised sui-

cide attempts. 2013.

17. Moore, A., Eternal sunshine, in The Guardian. 2007.

18. Shorter, E., A history of psychiatry: From the era of the asylum to the age of Prozac. 1997, New York: John Wiley & Sons.

19. Giliberti, M., Stand up for mental health care coverage. 2017, NAMI: email.

20. CDC, Table 51. Serious psychological distress in the past 30 days among adults aged 18 and over, by selected characteristics: United States, average annual, selected years 1997-1998 through 2012-2013. 1985, Centers for Disease Control and Prevention: Atlanta: GA.

21. Styron, W., Darkness visible: A memoir of madness. First edition. ed. 1990, New York Random House.

22. Barber, C., Comfortably numb: How psychiatry is medicating a nation. 2008, New York: Pantheon Books.

23. Kramer, P.D., Ordinarily well: The case for antidepressants. 2016, New York: Farrar, Straus and Giroux.

24. Goethe, J.W.v., The sorrows of Young Werther, Elective affinities. 1902, Boston: F.A. Nicolls & Co.

25. Glenmullen, J., Prozac backlash: Overcoming the dangers of Prozac, Zoloft, Paxil, and other antidepressants with safe, effective alternatives. 2000, New York: Simon and Schuster.

26. Wilson, E., Against happiness: In praise of melancholy. 2008, New York: Farrar, Straus and Giroux.

27. Wurtzel, E., Prozac nation: Young and depressed in America. 1994, Boston: Houghton Mifflin.

28. Norden, M.J., Beyond Prozac: Brain-toxic lifestyles, natural antidotes & new generation antidepressants. 1995, New York: ReganBooks.

29. McCarthy, T., Review: "Prozac Nation". Variety, 2001.

30. Kakutani, M., The examined life is not worth living either, in The New York Times.

31. Glatt, C.R., Prozac Nation review. Library Journal, 1994. 119(13): p. 110.

32. Ryan, H.L., Normalizing happiness: The rhetoric of depression in direct-to-consumer advertising, in Dept. of English. 2009, University of Arizona. p. 1-173.

33. Slater, L., Prozac diary. 1998, New York: Penguin Books.

34. Berlin, R.M., ed. Poets on Prozac: Mental illness, treatment, and the creative process. 2008, The Johns Hopkins University Press: Baltimore.

35. Dworkin, R.W., Artificial happiness: The dark side of the new happy class. 2006, New York: Carroll & Graf.

36. Healy, D., Let them eat Prozac: The unhealthy relationship between the pharmaceutical industry and depression. 2004, New York: New York University Press.

37. Kramer, P.D., Listening to Prozac. 1997, New York: Penguin Books.

38. Sharpe, K., The silence of Prozac. Lancet Psychiatry, 2015. 2(10): p. 871-3.

39. Elliott, C., Better than well: American medicine meets the American dream. 2003, New York: W.W. Norton.

40. Edwards, J.C., Passion, activity, and the care of self: Foucault and Heidegger in the precincts of Prozac, in Prozac as a way of life, C. Elliott and T. Chambers, Editors. 2004, University of North Carolina Press: Chapel Hill.

41. DeGrazia, D., Prozac, enhancement, and self-creation, in Prozac as a way of life, C. Elliott and T. Chambers, Editors. 2004, University of North Carolina Press: Chapel Hill.

42. Kirmayer, L.J., The sound of one hand clapping: Listening to Prozac in Japan, in Prozac as a way of life, C. Elliott and T. Chambers, Editors. 2004, University of North Carolina Press: Chapel Hill.

43. Parens, E., Kramer's anxiety, in Prozac as a way of life, C.

Elliott and T. Chambers, Editors. 2004, University of North Carolina Press: Chapel Hill.

44. Elliott, C. and T. Chambers, eds. Prozac as a way of life. 2004, University of North Carolina Press: Chapel Hill.

45. Kramer, P.D., The valorization of sadness: Alienation and the melancholic temperament, in Prozac as a way of life, C. Elliott and T. Chambers, Editors. 2004, University of North Carolina Press: Chapel Hill.

46. CDC, 10 leading causes of death by age group, United States—2015. 2015, Centers for Disease Control and Prevention: Atlanta, GA.

47. Elliott, C., Pursued by happiness and beaten senseless: Prozac and the American dream, in Prozac as a way of life, C. Elliott and T. Chambers, Editors. 2004, University of North Carolina Press: Chapel Hill.

48. Zoloth, L., Care of the dying in America, in Prozac as a way of life, C. Elliott and T. Chambers, Editors. 2004, University of North Carolina Press: Chapel Hill.

49. Hacking, I., Rewriting the soul. 1995, Princeton, N.J.: Princeton University Press.

50. Trilling, L., Sincerity and authenticity. 1972, Cambridge, Mass.: Harvard University Press.

51. Healy, D., Good science or bad business?, in Prozac as a Way of Life, C. Elliott and T. Chambers, Editors. 2004, University of North Carolina Press: Chapel Hill.

52. Clay, R.A. The next DSM. Monitor on Psychology, 2013. 44.

53. APA, Diagnostic and statistical manual of mental disorders: DSM-I. 1952, Washington, DC: American Psychiatric Association.

54. WHO, Constitution of the World Health Organization. 2006, World Health Organization: Geneva.

55. WHO, Mental Health Action Plan 2013-2020. 2013, Gene-

va: World Health Organization.

56. Emmons, K.K., Black dogs and blue words. 2014, New Brunswick, NJ: Rutgers University Press.

57. Blazer, D., The age of melancholy. 2005, New York: Routledge.

58. Foucault, M., Madness and civilization: A history of insanity in the Age of Reason. 1965, New York: Random House.

59. van Praag, H.M., "Make-believes" in psychiatry. 1993, New York: Brunner/Mazel.

60. CDC, Table 86. Selected prescription drug classes used in the past 30 days, by sex and age: United States, selected years 1988-1994 through 2009-2012. n.d., Centers for Disease Control and Prevention: Atlanta: GA.

61. Nielsen, A.C. and T.A. Williams, Depression in ambulatory medical patients: Prevalence by self-report questionnaire and recognition by nonpsychiatric physicians. Archives of General Psychiatry, 1980. 37(9): p. 999-1004.

62. CMS, Table 01 National Health Expenditures and Selected Economic Indicators [2008–2014]. 2015, Centers for Medicare and Medicaid Services.

63. Rice, D.P., T.A. Hodgson, and A.N. Kopstein, The economic costs of illness: A replication and update. Health Care Finance Review, 1985. 7(1): p. 61-80.

64. Greenberg, P.E., et al., The economic burden of depression in the United States: How did it change between 1990 and 2000? The Journal of Clinical Psychiatry, 2003. 64(12): p. 1465-75.

65. APA Quantifying the cost of depression. Center for Workplace Mental Health, n.d.

66. Wong, D.T., K.W. Perry, and F.P. Bymaster, The discovery of fluoxetine hydrochloride (Prozac). Nature Reviews Drug Discovery, 2005. 4(9): p. 764-774.

67. Kessler, R.C., The costs of depression. The Psychiatric

Clinics of North America, 2012. 35(1): p. 1-14.

68. Knapp, M., Hidden costs of mental illness. The British Journal of Psychiatry, 2003. 183(6): p. 477-478.

69. Greenberg, P.E., et al., The economic burden of adults with major depressive disorder in the United States (2005 and 2010). The Journal of Clinical Psychiatry, 2015. 76(2): p. 155-62.

70. PwC Medical cost trend: Behind the numbers 2018. 2017.

71. CDC, Lack of health insurance coverage and type of coverage, earlyrelease201611_01.pdf, Editor. 2017, Centers for Disease Control and Prevention: Atlanta, GA.

72. Himmelstein, D. and S. Woolhandler, Repealing the Affordable Care Act will kill more than 43,000 people annually, in The Washington Post. 2017.

73. Hare, D.L., et al., Depression and cardiovascular disease: A clinical review. European Heart Journal, 2014. 35(21): p. 1365-72.

74. Helliwell, J., R. Layard, and J. Sachs World happiness report 2016. 2016.

75. Lohoff, F.W., Overview of the genetics of major depressive disorder. Current Psychiatry Reports, 2010. 12(6): p. 539-546.

76. Breen, G., et al., A genome-wide significant linkage for severe depression on chromosome 3: The depression network study. American Journal of Psychiatry, 2011. 168(8): p. 840-847.

77. Hillhouse, T.M. and J.H. Porter, A brief history of the development of antidepressant drugs: From monoamines to glutamate. Experimental and Clinical Psychopharmacology, 2015. 23(1): p. 1-21.

78. Hirschkop, P.J. and J.R. Mook, Revisiting the lessons of Osheroff v. Chestnut Lodge, in American Academy of Psychiatry and the Law. 2012: Montreal, Canada.

79. Walsh, M.T. and T.G. Dinan, Selective serotonin reuptake inhibitors and violence: a review of the available evidence. Acta Psychiatrica Scandinavica, 2001. 104(2): p. 84-91.

80. Bornstein, J.C., Serotonin in the gut: What does it do? Frontiers in Neuroscience, 2012. 6: p. 16.

81. Niciu, M.J., et al., Glutamate and its receptors in the pathophysiology and treatment of major depressive disorder. Journal of Neural Transmission, 2014. 121(8): p. 907-924.

82. Lilly, E., Prescribing information for Prozac, E. Lilly, Editor. 2017, Eli Lilly.

83. Jick, S.S., A.D. Dean, and H. Jick, Antidepressants and suicide. British Medical Journal, 1995. 310: p. 215-18.

84. Slater, L., Kafka's boys: A story of sex and serotonin, in Prozac as a way of life, C. Elliott and T. Chambers, Editors. 2004, University of North Carolina Press: Chapel Hill.

85. Olfson, M., et al., Antidepressant prescribing practices of outpatient psychiatrists. Archives of General Psychiatry, 1998. 55(4): p. 310-316.

86. Pincus, H., et al., Prescribing trends in psychotropic medications: Primary care, psychiatry, and other medical specialties. JAMA, 1998. 279(7): p. 526-531.

87. Miller, S.G. 1 in 6 Americans takes a psychiatric drug. Scientific American, 2016.

88. CCHR Mental health America. n.d.

89. MHA MHA annual report 2016. 2016.

90. NCHS, Health, United States, 2016: With chartbook on long-term trends in health, H.a.H. Services, Editor. 2016, National Center for Health Statistics: Hyattsville, MD.

91. CDC, National ambulatory medical care survey: 2014 state and national summary tables. 2014: Atlanta: GA.

92. Pratt, L.A., Brody, Debra J., & Gu, Qiuping, Antidepressant use in persons aged 12 and over: United States, 2005–2008. NCHS Data Brief, 2011. 76(October 2011).

93. Kantor, E.D., et al., Trends in prescription drug use among adults in the United States from 1999-2012. Journal of the Ameri-

can Medical Association, 2015. 314(17): p. 1818-1830.

94. Leonard, M., Are children the hot new market for antidepressants?, in The Boston Globe. 1997.

95. Kesselheim, A.S., J. Avorn, and A. Sarpatwari, The high cost of prescription drugs in the United States: Origins and prospects for reform. Journal of the American Medical Association, 2016. 316(8): p. 858-871.

96. GoodRX. SSRIs. 2017; Available from: https://www.goodrx.com/ssris.

97. APA, Diagnostic and statistical manual of mental disorders : DSM-2. 1968, Washington, DC: American Psychiatric Association.

98. Klerman, G.L., et al., Neurotic depressions: A systematic analysis of multiple criteria and meanings. American Journal of Psychiatry, 1979. 136(1): p. 57-61.

99. Rosenhan, D.L., On being sane in insane places. Clinical Social Work Journal, 1974. 2(4): p. 237-256.

100. APA, Diagnostic and statistical manual of mental disorders : DSM-5. 5th ed. 2013, Arlington: VA: American Psychiatric Association.

101. Szasz, T., The manufacture of madness: A comparative study of the inquisition and the mental health movement. 1970, New York: Harper & Row.

102. MHA Mental health in America—Prevalence data. 2018.

103. Squier, S., The paradox of Prozac as an enhancement technology, in Prozac as a way of life, C. Elliott and T. Chambers, Editors. 2004, University of North Carolina Press: Chapel Hill.

104. NIMH Just over half of Americans diagnosed with major depression receive care. Science News, 2010.

105. Gøtzsche, P.C., A.H. Young, and J. Crace, Does long term use of psychiatric drugs cause more harm than good? British Medical Journal, 2015. 350.

106. Whitaker, J. Mental health screening. 2018.

107. Kirsch, I. and G. Sapirstein, Listening to Prozac but hearing placebo: A meta-analysis of antidepressant medications, in How expectancies shape experience, I. Kirsch, Editor. 1999, American Psychological Association: Washington, DC.

108. FDA, Prozac® fluoxetine hydrochloride description. 2004.

109. FDA, Updates: Prozac for pediatric use. FDA Consumer, 2003(March-April 2003).

110. CDC Childrens' mental health: Anxiety and depression. 2017.

111. FDA, Suicidality in children and adolescents being treated with antidepressant medications. 2004, U.S. Food and Drug Administration.

112. Keller, M.B., et al., A multi-center, double-blind, placebo controlled study of paroxetine and imipramine in adolescents with unipolar major depression. 2001, SmithKline Beecham.

113. Carey, B., Antidepressant Paxil is unsafe for teenagers, new analysis says, in The New York Times. 2015.

114. Doshi, P., Putting GlaxoSmithKline to the test over paroxetine. British Medical Journal, 2013. 347.

115. Le Noury, J., et al., Restoring Study 329: Efficacy and harms of paroxetine and imipramine in treatment of major depression in adolescence. British Medical Journal, 2015. 351.

116. Teicher, M.H., C. Glod, and J.O. Cole, Emergence of intense suicidal preoccupation during fluoxetine treatment. American Journal of Psychiatry, 1990. 147(2): p. 207-10.

117. Mann, J. and S. Kapur, The emergence of suicidal ideation and behavior during antidepressant pharmacotherapy. Archives of General Psychiatry, 1991. 48(11): p. 1027-1033.

118. Donovan, S., et al., Deliberate self-harm and antidepressant drugs. British Journal of Psychiatry, 2000. 177(6): p. 551-556.

119. Friedman, R.A., Antidepressants' Black-Box Warning—10 Years Later. New England Journal of Medicine, 2014. 371(18): p. 1666-1668.

120. FDA, Revisions to product labeling. 2007, Food and Drug Administration.

121. Ventola, C.L., Direct-to-consumer pharmaceutical advertising: Therapeutic or toxic? Pharmacy and Therapeutics, 2011. 36(10): p. 669-684.

122. NIHCM Prescription drugs and mass media advertising. Research Brief, 2000.

123. Heifferon, B. and S.C. Brown, Guest Editor's Column. Technical Communication Quarterly, 2000. 9: p. 245-48.

124. Rosenthal, M.B., et al., Promotion of Prescription Drugs to Consumers. New England Journal of Medicine, 2002. 346(7): p. 498-505.

125. Gross, A.G., The rhetoric of science. 1996, Cambridge: Harvard University.

126. Fahnestock, J., Accommodating science: The rhetorical life of scientific facts. Written Communication, 1986. 3(3): p. 275-296.

127. States, U., Prescription Drugs: Improvements Needed in FDA's Oversight of Direct-to-Consumer Advertising, G.A. Office, Editor. 2006: Washington, D.C.

128. Lewis, G., Dark gifts, in Poets on Prozac: Mental illness, treatment, and the creative process, R.M. Berlin, Editor. 2008, The Johns Hopkins University Press: Baltimore.

129. Lefcowitz, B.F., From bog to crystal, in Poets on Prozac: Mental illness, treatment, and the creative process, R.M. Berlin, Editor. 2008, The Johns Hopkins University Press: Baltimore.

130. Chambers, T., Prozac for the sick soul, in Prozac as a way of life, C. Elliott and T. Chambers, Editors. 2004, University of North Carolina Press: Chapel Hill.

131. Powell, R., My name is not Alice, in Poets on Prozac: Mental illness, treatment, and the creative process, R.M. Berlin, Editor. 2008, The Johns Hopkins University Press: Baltimore.

132. Smith, J.D., The desire to think clearly, in Poets on Prozac: Mental illness, treatment, and the creative process, R.M. Berlin, Editor. 2008, The Johns Hopkins University Press: Baltimore.

133. Porter, L., Down the tracks: Bruce Springsteen sang to me, in Poets on Prozac: Mental illness, treatment, and the creative process, R.M. Berlin, Editor. 2008, The Johns Hopkins University Press: Baltimore.

134. Coulehan, J., In the middle of life's journey, in Poets on Prozac: Mental illness, treatment, and the creative process, R.M. Berlin, Editor. 2008, The Johns Hopkins University Press: Baltimore.

135. Krampf, T., Perfecting the art of falling, in Poets on Prozac: Mental illness, treatment, and the creative process, R.M. Berlin, Editor. 2008, The Johns Hopkins University Press: Baltimore.

136. Ashley, R., Depression and the ordinary, in Poets on Prozac: Mental Illness, Treatment, and the Creative Process, R.M. Berlin, Editor. 2008, The Johns Hopkins University Press: Baltimore.

137. Eppolito, C., Food for thought, in Poets on Prozac: Mental illness, treatment, and the creative process, R.M. Berlin, Editor. 2008, The Johns Hopkins University Press: Baltimore.

138. Haley, V., How I learned to count to four and live with the ghosts of animals, in Poets on Prozac: Mental illness, treatment, and the creative process, R.M. Berlin, Editor. 2008, The Johns Hopkins University Press: Baltimore.

139. Budbill, D., The uses of depression: The way around is through, in Poets on Prozac: Mental illness, treatment, and the

creative process, R.M. Berlin, Editor. 2008, The Johns Hopkins University Press: Baltimore.

140. Millner, J., My oldest voice, in Poets on Prozac: Mental illness, treatment, and the creative process, R.M. Berlin, Editor. 2008, The Johns Hopkins University Press: Baltimore.

141. Rothenberg, A., Creativity and madness: New findings and old stereotypes. 1990, Baltimore, MD: Johns Hopkins University Press.

142. White, J., Summers off. Crazyhorse, 2016(90): p. 8-17.

143. Sarraute, N., Martereau: A novel. 2004, Champaign, IL: Dalkey Archive Press.

144. Eliot, T.S., The sacred wood: Essays on poetry and criticism. 1932, London: Methuen.

145. Joyce, J., A portrait of the artist as a young man. 2005, London: CRW Publishing.

146. Mann, K., The turning point: Thirty-five years in this century, the autobiography of Klaus Mann. 1942, New York: L.B. Fischer.

147. Diekstra, R.F., The epidemiology of suicide and parasuicide. Acta Psychiatrica Scandinavica Suppl, 1993. 371: p. 9-20.

148. CDC/NCHS, Leading causes of death and numbers of deaths, by sex, race, and Hispanic origin: United States, 1980 and 2014, https://www.cdc.gov/nchs/data/hus/2015/019.pdf, Editor. 2014, Public Health Service: Washington, DC.

149. CDC, National Vital Statistics Reports, 2016. 64(2): p. 1-118.

150. CDC, Number of deaths for leading causes of death. FastStats, 2016.

151. Vijayakumar, L., Suicide in women. Indian Journal of Psychiatry, 2015. 57(Suppl 2): p. S233-S238.

152. Wiley, Paxil use: New warnings for young adults. Mental Health Weekly, 2016(19 Jun 2016).

153. Fava, M. and J.F. Rosenbaum, Suicidality and fluoxetine: Is there a relationship? The Journal of Clinical Psychiatry, 1991. 52(3): p. 108-111.

154. Dete, T.P. and H.G. Jarecki, Modern psychiatric treatment. 1971, Philadelphia: J.B. Lippincott.

155. Beasley, C.M.J., et al., Fluoxetine and suicide: A meta-analysis of controlled trials of treatment for depression. International Clinical Psychopharmacology, 1992. 6: p. 35-57.

156. Donovan, S., et al., The occurrence of suicide following the prescription of antidepressant drugs. Archives of Suicide Research, 1999. 5(3): p. 181-192.

157. Beck, A.T., et al., Hopelessness and eventual suicide: A 10-year prospective study of patients hospitalized with suicidal ideation. American Journal of Psychiatry, 1985. 142(5): p. 559-63.

158. Elkin, I., et al., National Institute of Mental Health Treatment of Depression Collaborative Research Program. General effectiveness of treatments. Archives of General Psychiatry, 1989. 46(11): p. 971-82; discussion 983.

159. Persons, J.B., J. Davidson, and M.A. Tompkins, Essential components of cognitive-behavior therapy for depression. 2000, Washington, DC: American Psychological Association.

160. Goldman, M.S., Expectancy operation: Cognitive-neural models and architectures, in How expectancies shape experience, I. Kirsch, Editor. 1999, American Psychological Association: Washington, DC.

www.ingramcontent.com/pod-product-compliance
Lightning Source LLC
Chambersburg PA
CBHW052056110526
44591CB00013B/2233